FLOWERS IN THE DARK

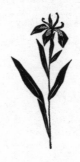

ALSO BY SISTER DANG NGHIEM

Healing: A Woman's Journey from Doctor to Nun

Mindfulness as Medicine: A Story of Healing Body and Spirit

FLOWERS *in* *the* DARK

Reclaiming Your Power to Heal from Trauma with Mindfulness

SISTER DANG NGHIEM, MD

PARALLAX PRESS
BERKELEY, CALIFORNIA

PARALLAX PRESS

P.O. Box 7355
Berkeley, California 94707
parallax.org

Parallax Press is the publishing division of Plum Village Community
of Engaged Buddhism, Inc.

Cover and text design by Katie Eberle
Cover photo by Yousef Espanioly
Some names and identifying details have been changed to protect the privacy
of individuals.

Content warning: This book contains material that readers may find triggering,
including references to self-harm, sexual abuse, and trauma.

Disclaimer: The following information is intended for general information
purposes only. Individuals should always see their health-care provider before
administering any suggestions made in this book. All matters regarding mental
health require medical supervision. Neither the publisher nor the author is
engaged in rendering professional advice to the individual reader. Neither the
author nor the publisher shall be liable or responsible for any loss or damage
allegedly arising from any information or suggestion in this book. Any application
of the material set forth in the following pages is at the reader's discretion and is
his or her sole responsibility.

Printed in the United States of America on FSC Certified paper.
Library of Congress Cataloging-in-Publication Data is available on request.

3 4 5 / 24 23 22

To my beloved teacher, Zen Master Thich Nhat Hanh
Thanks to your guidance, love, and trust, my healing
and this book become possible.

To my editor, Hisae, with thanks for your faith and dedication

For those of us who have been a victim of sexual abuse, there is a teaching that we have learned—that the mud and the lotus inter-are. It is possible to transform the mud into the lotus. Everything is impermanent; everything changes.

—THICH NHAT HANH, IN A DHARMA TALK AT
PLUM VILLAGE, FRANCE, JUNE 16, 2009

CONTENTS

Look, my love, look at the innumerable flowers and leaves.

Look, my love, look at yourself,

Your wonderful manifestations are all these.

The spring is coming, from the heart of the winter.

The inspiration to write this book came to me at the end of a retreat I had taught in Atlanta, Georgia, in 2017. The organizers invited my monastic sisters and me to come to a garden behind their church to see the evening primroses bloom that night. Admittedly, I was not enthusiastic at the prospect since I was already quite tired after a long day at the retreat. Out of a sense of gratitude to our hosts, I still showed up.

At eight o'clock, about ten of us gathered in the church garden around the long stems of a tall, slender plant covered in drying, wilted yellow flowers. A friend of mine began to pluck away these old flowers, so that the new blossoms, indicated by tightly furled, spike-like buds, would be more visible to us. I stood politely, quiet and patient for what seemed like an interminable length of time. It began to get dark. Nothing seemed to happen. Suddenly, although there was no wind, the entire plant began to vibrate and tremble before us. Lo and behold, a flower bud suddenly and forcefully burst open, the petals unfolding one by one and then all at once, simultaneously, right in front of my eyes. This entire process took place within the space of a breath!

My mouth fell open and tears began streaming down my cheeks. As a somewhat poetic-minded lover of literature, I had often talked about flowers bursting into bloom; I had sung songs about them, written poetry about them, and mentioned them in Dharma talks, cleverly using the metaphor to make my points. Yet in that moment, on that day in front of this evening primrose plant, I woke up to the fact that I had never directly experienced how a flower actually blooms! Seeing these delicate yellow flowers spring open in the darkness awoke in me the realization that healing from trauma—recovering from painful experiences so that we can flourish and grow—is both simple and miraculous, a process that will unfold naturally, when enough of the right conditions are present.

For thirty years of my life, I had seen myself as a victim, isolated in my suffering. The facts of my upbringing and life story are now known—I've written about them in a memoir and frequently mentioned them in public talks, and I recount some parts in this book as well. Less well known are the steps I've taken since I took refuge as a Buddhist nun, to heal from my past of childhood sexual abuse. When I ordained as a nun in 2000, I learned from my beloved teacher, Zen Master Thich Nhat Hanh, a teaching that I have found to be invaluable in my healing process: the "inner child" within us. "Thay," as his students address him (an affectionate word for "teacher" in Vietnamese) says,

> *In each of us, there is a young, suffering child. We have all had times of difficulty as children, and many of us have experienced trauma. To protect and defend ourselves against future suffering, we often try to forget those painful times. Every time we're in touch with the experience of suffering, we believe we can't bear it, and so we stuff our feelings and memories deep down in our unconscious mind. It may be that we haven't dared to face this child for many decades.*

Thich Nhat Hanh offers us a practice of saying hello and talking to our inner child. Combined with mindfulness training, the steady schedule, and the peaceful monastery ambiance, this practice slowly brought me back to life. The inner child practice Thich Nhat Hanh teaches is just one exercise among many in a holistic system of activities his tradition offers to the world for transforming pain and suffering—and generating peace and joy.

After the severe trauma I had undergone, I was able to connect with myself and heal by practicing mindfulness. Over the years, as I became a Dharma teacher in Thich Nhat Hanh's tradition, known as the Plum Village Community of Engaged Buddhism, many young people have come to me for counseling and I have taught them the same practices and walked together with them, privileged to witness their healing. You don't have to take monastic vows to benefit from mindfulness; you can start to benefit right away, wherever you are.

Thich Nhat Hanh has taught, "The only way for you to transform the pain as a victim of sexual abuse is to become a bodhisattva. You take a vow to aspire to protect individuals, couples, families, and children from sexual abuse. In this way, you become a bodhisattva. And when the bodhisattva energy is in you, the suffering of being a victim of sexual abuse will begin to dissolve." A bodhisattva is an ideal of a person who not only becomes enlightened for themselves, but also for others; they are an embodiment of compassion. Of course, not everyone who was abused will aspire to become a bodhisattva or even a spiritually oriented person, but this teaching can help anyone to take a step on a path of compassion, starting with self-compassion toward their inner child and radiating outward in their speech, thoughts, and actions toward others. Thich Nhat Hanh's words gave me the strength and inspiration to live my life as a healer.

In recent years, looking back at my journal entries as a young woman, I saw that even before meeting Thich Nhat Hanh, I had been able to name and acknowledge the "wounded child" inside me. In my journals and poems, I had written of my deep yearning to heal myself from my childhood pain and to protect young people from abuse. The wisdom and the aspiration had always been there, in the midst of suffering, but I simply did not know then how to realize them in this life, in each and every moment. Within each wounded child is a bodhisattva waiting for sufficient conditions to bloom.

Everyone suffering from trauma also has within them the capacity to heal, but they may not know it, and they may have obstacles to accessing their inner wisdom. In a culture of silence and shame, we survivors of sexual abuse may find it impossible to speak or even think about it, due to denial within the family or community. It takes a lot of courage for survivors to start on the path of healing and finally face our trauma. The reality is that it can be a long journey to find the resources we need to fully recover. The criminal justice system can address only limited aspects of individual and community healing, and assault victims frequently find such procedures retraumatizing. Professional therapy and counseling are needed as well, but access is not always easy. However, at a deep level we can always tap into our own embodied wisdom through practicing mindfulness in our daily lives, which brings about the deepest transformation and healing.

In this book, I wish to share the practices I have found most helpful on the journey to healing. We will see how mindfulness practice provides a bridge to our inner wisdom and calms the mind and nervous system. We will come to know our inner child and befriend them. These practices are helpful not only for survivors of childhood trauma, but for anyone troubled by trauma of any kind. We will look at some of the physiological and psychological aspects of trauma, as it is vital to understand how trauma affects our body, mind, and memory, and what we Buddhists call our "store consciousness" and "habit energy"—what psychologists call our subconscious mind.

In Buddhist psychology, we often talk about the Five Faculties, which with practice develop into the Five Strengths—trust, energy or diligence, mindfulness, concentration, and insight or wisdom. Of these factors, mindfulness is the foundation. In the central part of this book, we will look at how we can bring the Five Strengths into our everyday lives to help us on the path of healing. I will offer teachings for trauma survivors on these deep sources of inner empowerment. In addition to the basic Plum Village practices of mindful breathing, sitting, walking, and eating, I will invite you to explore the Five Strengths through some simple body-based meditations.

The Five Strengths work in sequence: trusting in ourselves and the healing process empowers us to take action, which in turn makes it possible to be mindful. Mindfulness leads to deep concentration, which gives rise to profound insight or wisdom, which frees us from the past. Wisdom is the greatest power of all. It guides and sustains us through even the most difficult times by giving us the right view and the skill to work through challenging circumstances in a way that fosters joy and freedom.

The Five Strengths are powerful friends on the path because they are the antidotes to their opposites. Trust heals doubt; diligence or energy transforms depression and apathy; mindfulness subdues impulsiveness and recklessness; concentration dispels distraction and avoidance; and insight or wisdom removes fear and hatred. As you develop the Five Strengths, even moderately, your mind begins to be freed from negative energies, and compassion and understanding can flourish. You find more peace in your life, and you learn to avoid chaos and drama.

The Five Strengths are one of several sets of qualities that Buddhist psychology offers as a holistic system for awakening, which we can intentionally cultivate to free ourselves from suffering. As an invitation to explore further, we'll look at how the five main Buddhist precepts support healing from trauma, as expressed in the Plum Village tradition's Five Mindfulness Trainings—Reverence for Life, True

Happiness, True Love, Loving Speech and Deep Listening, and Nourishment and Healing. You do not have to become a Buddhist to benefit from these trainings. In fact, people from many faiths or no faith at all can follow them, because Buddhism, at its root, is not a religion, but a practical approach to the art of living. Thich Nhat Hanh would often say, "Buddhism is not a religion but a practice."

Through this book, I hope you will gain an understanding of how mindfulness can be a powerful source of energy for your healing process. It is my deep wish that those suffering from post-traumatic stress, particularly survivors of sexual abuse like myself, have access to as many resources as possible. The practice of meditation is not meant to be a substitute for therapy with trained professionals, but if followed correctly, this path transforms suffering into true peace, happiness, and freedom. For myself, I have found that walking this path has helped me when other approaches could not. After all, as the example of the Buddha and two and a half millennia of practice demonstrate, if we follow the path wholeheartedly, with proper guidance, it can lead us to complete freedom from every type of suffering.

Mindfulness is a miracle because it enables us to behold ourselves and our lives as if we are witnessing the blossoming of a flower for the very first time. This sense of awe and wonder can help us heal past trauma and renew our life, moment to moment, in the most truthful, beautiful, and wholesome way. It is in this spirit that I am about to share with you the path to healing trauma that many beloved friends and I have personally traveled. May my telling of our experiences help you give voice to your experiences. May our transformation and healing be your own inspiration and realization.

SISTER DANG NGHIEM
DEER PARK MONASTERY, OCTOBER 2020

PART 1

TRAUMA *and* HEALING

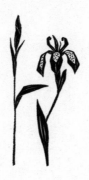

CHAPTER 1

Spanning the Bridge of Mindfulness

Refugees

Dragging their dark

Bodies, thin as fibrous

Roots, wearied as torn

Leaves, under the blade of

The reaper, they search

For sanctuary.

It was 1968. Bombs exploded all around, raining clods of dirt amidst the fire and smoke. Injured bodies writhed in the burning air. Those who still could were crawling and running underground through secret tunnels. My mother was in labor in one of these tunnels, being carried away hurriedly on an improvised stretcher by two farmers. In the midst of my mother's screams and the sound of conflict, I came to life, bloody and mute. My grandmother slapped my buttocks to make me cry. Thus, my life officially began, in suffering, yet nevertheless I was a fortunate survivor.

I was born in Central Vietnam during the Tet Offensive, the child of my Vietnamese mother and an American father whom I would never meet. There was heavy fighting in our area at the time. Soon after I was born, bombs dropped on our village and destroyed our home.

War brings chaos and the breakdown of boundaries. Human beings commit unspeakable atrocities, brothers fight brothers, and men violate women and girls. The pain and trauma of war continues, even when conditions are quieter on the surface. After the fall of Saigon in 1975, my mother, my younger brother, and I moved into a big house there to live with my mother's lover, whom we called "the old dad," who was thirty years older than my mother, about the same age as my grandmother. He became our provider, and, thankfully, he was safe to be around.

My uncle moved into the big house to live with us about a year later. He was my mother's younger brother by only a few years, so he would have been in his late twenties. He looked as if he were half-French with his curly light brown hair, fair skin, and Roman nose. Young women blushed and became shy in his presence.

I do not remember the first time he abused me, nor how many times it happened, nor how it happened. I was nine years old. I just remember having this repetitive, haunting thought in my mind: *I do not want to go with him again!* I would see myself walking up the staircase to the third floor and dreading every step of it. I would see myself sitting in the small bathroom up there, on a cement floor so cold and coarse it nipped at my skin. I would see my uncle naked right in front of me, his legs opened wide apart like a pair of tongs. His hands would reach out to grab my hand and place it on his penis. Everything took place like in a silent movie, with me being mute and frozen. My body did not seem to exist, except for my camera-like eyes, flickering, taking occasional snapshots, then closing, shutting everything out.

My mother's dream was to go to America, and all she thought about was leaving. She was not aware of the sexual abuse that I was going through, and she herself was physically and verbally violent toward me. One day in May in 1980, my mother went out to the market as usual, but she never came back. A naked body wrapped inside plastic and coarse cloth was found floating on a river near our house, but my grandmother and my aunt could not determine whether it was my mother's body, since it was severely swollen. She was thirty-six, and I was twelve. At first, I was secretly happy and relieved by her disappearance, because I would then no longer have to endure her kicks and blows. I remember thinking, "Good, from now on she will not abuse me anymore!"

My grandmother became the sole person to raise my brother, Sonny, and me. When she felt we were old enough, she sent us to the United States via an amnesty program for Amerasian children from the war. It was 1985. My grandmother said we were going to America for a better future. She insisted that I should take good care of my brother, get a higher education, and eventually become a Buddhist nun.

I did accomplish all those things. My brother and I remain close to this day, I earned not one but two bachelor's degrees and then an MD, and at the time of this writing I have been a Buddhist nun for more than twenty years. Grandma passed away in 1986, a year after Sonny and I left Vietnam, but to this day I still feel her daily presence helping and protecting me in my spiritual life. Those of us with childhood trauma might have had parents who abused us or failed to protect us. If we are lucky, we may also have had at least one person in our lives—for me, it was my grandmother—who can transmit to us a sense of unconditional love, which can literally save our lives.

While growing up in the United States, I experienced so much hardship and despair that I often wanted to take my own life. Then the image of my grandmother would come back to me in my dreams, sitting still on her hard wooden bed and praying to the Buddha. I would wake up in the middle of the night to a feeling of restored peace. And in the morning, I would feel reinvigorated enough to get up, wash my face, change my clothes, and move forward in my day. Later, when I was in college, I wrote the following poem about her.

GRANDMA

Once I asked if you loved me. You laughed and questioned who would love my dog-born face. Then you turned away to cough, and I awkwardly reached for your back. Once I kissed your cheeks and tasted grooves of your skin between my lips. You hit my teenage pimple with your quivering fist. I laughed and dabbed my tears.

And the day I left you for America, you placed my hands in your spread-out palm. You spit chewed betel juice and circled it slowly on my hands, saying, "This is to help you not to miss Grandma too much." You refused to go to the airport.

I was sixteen and a half when I left Viet Nam with a five-dollar bill and a few English greeting phrases. From America, I wanted to send you newspapers and Smitty's plastic bags, so you could sell them by the gram; people threw them away here. I wanted to send you a waterbed, so you could float gently to your sleep; your seventy-five-year-old body would not have to strike against the wooden plank bed anymore. I worked the midnight shift at a post office to send you dollars, bars of soap, white laces, bottles of green oil.

I did not send you medicine, but prayers. Every night, I prayed for
you, while I listened to the echo of your constant coughing, of
the hard thumps against your aching body. The day I heard you
died, I looked at my face, half belonging to my mother, half to an
unknown man, and I cried with a fist, yours, in my mouth.

An orphan carrying invisible wounds from my childhood, I arrived in the United States as a sixteen-year-old refugee, holding the hand of my twelve-year-old brother. We were sent to live in Tempe, Arizona. My younger brother and I bounced from one foster home to another, but I focused on my studies, taking refuge in academic achievement. (This, as we will see, is a common pattern with people with trauma: we keep ourselves busy to avoid our feelings.) I wrote poetry and journaled, and I was lucky to have teachers in my life who paid attention and supported me toward higher education. After working my way through a bachelor of arts degree in creative writing and a bachelor of science degree in psychology, I left Arizona to train as a physician at the University of California, San Francisco School of Medicine (UCSF). I went into family practice. I volunteered as an intern in Kenya and in India. I was a true immigrant success story. I had a respected position in society, money, an apartment in San Francisco, and a loving relationship with an extraordinary, wonderful man, John.

Soon after I started working as a doctor, I attended a mindfulness retreat with Zen Master Thich Nhat Hanh, whom I would come to address as "Thay," my "teacher" in Vietnamese. At the retreat, I woke up to the true state of my life. I had believed that after all the hardships I had been through, I would be happy if I had a good job and a beautiful, loving relationship. Like many survivors of trauma, I naively believed that working insanely hard and achieving success would make up for my past misfortunes. To my surprise, this was not the case. I had everything I wanted, but I was inexorably haunted by my past. I continued to behave as if I were still a little girl, wounded and confused. This discombobulated child manifested in my daily life through my thinking, my speech, and my behaviors, and it hurt my relationships, especially with John.

Suffering was alive and well in me. When we are children, many things happen to us, pleasant and unpleasant, and we don't have control over those conditions. Even when the original causes and conditions of our traumas are no longer present, we may still continue to suffer. As an educated young woman, I didn't have anyone treating me badly. Yet my way of thinking, speaking, and behaving caused me to perpetuate my own suffering in many ways. It was as if I subconsciously kept my trauma alive and fed it. I struggled with feelings of unworthiness, which affected my relationship with John. Despite going to medical school and absorbing the scientific approach to the mind through psychiatry and psychotherapy, I had no way of getting in touch with my suffering and the wounded child within me.

At this first retreat, I realized that the causes and conditions of my suffering were now no longer external, but internal. That was the first time I recognized that the way out of suffering was to turn my attention inward. "The way out is *in*," Thay liked to say. I needed to come back to myself and no longer point the finger outward looking for external causes. These insights were born from my first steps on the path of mindfulness.

Childhood trauma has the most severe impact, but even when we are adults, things that occur outside our control can still cause trauma. Three weeks after this first retreat, on the day before my birthday, my beloved John died. He had been seen at the beach in Half Moon

Bay where he sometimes swam. He never came back to his car, and his clothes sat unclaimed on the beach until some people noticed and alerted the coast guard. I received the news at 2 a.m., while I was on call at the Oakland Children's Hospital.

John's sudden death seemed to wake up every single cell of my body. He had loved life so much and he had lived so fully, with such lightness and tenderness, that when he died I honestly believed that he had nothing to regret. My own spirit, however, was broken. I could not go back to my old life, because the suffering that had been filling me to the brim was now spilling over. I did not have the capacity to continue living as before. I faced two stark choices: one was to end my life and the other was to take refuge in the teachings of the Buddha and transform my suffering completely.

I saw clearly that if I ended my life by my own hand, all the good and beautiful things I knew to be true—all the seeds of hope and confidence that I had planted in my brother and the young people I knew—would never compensate for the pain and confusion my death would cause them. I thought about my brother, the only family I had. I thought about the patients and the incarcerated youth I had cared for during the six years of my medical training. This sense of responsibility to them somehow saved me.

The path of spiritual practice was my only real option. Within three months of John's death, I had joined Thich Nhat Hanh and his community in the Plum Village monastery in rural southwest France. First founded as a home for refugees by Thich Nhat Hanh and peace activist and social worker Sister Chan Khong, Plum Village is now a home for several hundred monks and nuns. It was the right environment for me to learn how to meditate, transform my suffering, and give time to my healing process.

Interbeing

*"To be" is to inter-be. You cannot just be by yourself alone. You have to
inter-be with every other thing.*

—THICH NHAT HANH

Mindfulness practice rests on key teachings from Buddhist psychology
about the mind, as well as the interconnectedness of experience and
time. Everyone who undergoes severe trauma faces similar choices: to
try to pick up the pieces of our lives and continue as before; or to stop
and turn more intentionally toward healing, however that may appear
in our lives. While we may not recognize it at the time of a traumatic
event, life-changing suffering has a way of being an opening to a greater
understanding of life.

The "mud" and mess of our most painful experiences can become
the fertile ground for the blossoming of our understanding and
self-compassion. This is a hard truth to accept if we are resolved to
see a good life as consisting only of positive events. It is true that the
cool waters of happiness are sweet and precious, but it is suffering that
carves our cup.

The Buddha's Four Noble Truths acknowledge that life contains
suffering within it—but it is exactly this suffering that causes us to
seek a way out. If the war in Vietnam had not happened, my father,
an American soldier, would never have met my mother, and I would
never have been born. Thich Nhat Hanh would never have gone into
exile and never would have founded the Plum Village practice centers
in France. Without the upheaval and violence of the war, Thich Nhat
Hanh's teachings of peace and mindfulness would not have taken root
in the West. Within the worst sorrows may lie the greatest joys, and

the opposite may also be true. This happened because that happened; this is because that is; every event is interrelated in a web of causality, everything coming into being together. This is *interbeing*.

We cannot have the lotus without mud. We cannot have roses without the rain. This knowledge of interbeing helps us see the mud with new eyes. When there is trauma involving another person, we may try to cut off the pain by breaking off contact with them. This may be difficult if they are a family member, but it is possible. What is not possible is to separate ourselves from the perpetrator within us. We may change our outer circumstances and try to forget the people and situations that caused us to suffer, but they continue to live within us and disturb us, sometimes relentlessly.

Changing our perspective on our suffering helps us respond to it differently. Change is hard to put into practice, however. We are creatures of habit, after all. Meditation is a process of waking up from living on autopilot, so that we can choose a different approach to how we look at our world, and how we react to our perceptions. Changing our mind isn't only an intellectual or metaphysical exercise. Changing our mind about our trauma affects every aspect of ourselves, because as we now know, the mind and body *inter-are*. What happens to one affects the other. By meditating and following the path of mindfulness, we will experience moments of insight that open up space in our lives for healing. Similarly, because we are social beings, we find that what happens to one person in our community affects us all, in one way or another.

Healing the Present Heals the Past and the Future

In Buddhism, the three times of past, present, and future are not linear. They are in each other, true to the spirit of interbeing. The present contains the past because the past caused the present. The present also contains the future, because the future is determined by how we handle the present moment. This means that the past also contains the present and future, because the seeds of the present and future were there then. Just as a tree's limbs keep on branching at each point, so that they follow an infinitely repeating fractal pattern, this metaphor of branching and interdependent origination can help us understand how a traumatic moment can be factored into and enmeshed with subsequent moments as well as previous moments in life. It is this intricately connecting pattern that also enables healing in the now to infuse previous as well as future moments with healing.

The insight of interbeing also taught me that the traumatic experiences I went through are not mine alone. We do not have to curl up in a corner with our pain. The revelations of interbeing can inspire us and empower us to heal ourselves, because we know that when one person heals, that person helps many others in society to heal as well. We are fractal structures of our society. We do not heal in isolation; our healing is collective.

When we learn to work skillfully with our suffering, we are not only helping ourselves, we are also showing others that there is a way out of their own hurt. This principle of interbeing applies inside of us too. The wounds of both the victims and perpetrators within us will benefit from our practice and we become stronger and more resilient.

So, we lay down a path on the ground, stone by stone. When we come to a fast-flowing, dangerous river, we lay down a bridge. In our families and communities, there are currents of ancestral trauma—sometimes strongly flowing, sometimes underground and hidden, erupting when certain conditions arise. When we become aware of such collective traumas, we can see them as an opportunity to take care of suffering, not only for ourselves but also for others who may cross the bridge after us. Then many people after us will be able to cross that bridge without having to fall into the violent stream.

Mindfulness is the bridge that helps us arrive at the other side safely. It allows us to bring about the transformation of suffering into healing, insight, and wisdom. We can be a bodhisattva and take it as our aspiration to protect individuals, couples, families, and children from sexual abuse. The awareness and understanding that many others also need to find a way out has inspired me to practice and to heal myself, so I can help others do the same. It can be hard at times to believe that there is a way out of suffering, that happiness is possible and the way to it can be found. Yes, intergenerational trauma is real, but it is also true that generations of practitioners have lovingly tended a path that can lead us out of our suffering and into a peaceful and joyful life—just as the path was tended for them, century after century.

The garden grows the gardener. We can practice in our daily life to transform the suffering in us, and to harvest the wholesome and fulfilling elements that are within and around us every day. In life there are not only flowers, but also thorns, weeds, and decaying matter. Still, vibrant flowers flourish everywhere. No matter what stage of transformation our garden is at, we may still rest under the trees, enjoying the cool breeze, the shade, and the peace that comes with relishing life's simple pleasures.

Meditation as a Daily Source of Nourishment

Since becoming a nun, I have found ways of generating healing for the pain I encountered in my life before ordaining. Together with the understanding of how the brain processes trauma, the Buddhist approach to suffering can bring vitality back to frozen areas of the body and the mind with practices for increasing awareness of the breath and body.

You might think that meditation is a process of constantly confronting and combating your suffering and pain. But trauma survivor or not, it is important for us to find peace, joy, and happiness in the practice. In fact, the joy of meditation is a necessary daily nourishment to the spiritual practitioner.

Most of the time, we meditate simply to enjoy being fully alive, and we sit simply to enjoy our sitting and breathing with a relaxed body, the way a gardener enjoys planting seeds, watering flowers, and marveling at their intricacies and subtleties. Meditation is to be present for life, which is here and now. Meditation is to see clearly into something, and thus we gain deep insight into our happiness and suffering. Meditation is to bring light into something—that's why we use the word "enlightenment"—so that the layers of harmful perceptions and old views can be sloughed off and the barriers removed. That is why we use the word "enlightenment"—we are opening our eyes and waking up to the way things are.

In this book, you will learn some simple but powerful meditations for trauma, which will guide you to apply mindfulness to your suffering and gain insights that can heal both body and mind. Meditation is a process of self-discovery, but it must be grounded in genuine self-love for it to be healing. Ultimately, combined with the other elements of the path, meditation should help you establish peace in your mind and body. It is a way out of suffering.

A word of caution. If you have experienced post-traumatic stress, please proceed slowly, to avoid retriggering trauma. With the right guidance, mindfulness increases survivors' sense of safety and stability in daily life, as well as in challenging moments. As you have consciously chosen to read this book, I know that you are committed to your healing. But please be gentle with yourself. Never push yourself. I am not prescribing practices to be followed without questioning. If any of them feel unhelpful or uncomfortable, don't make yourself do them. Your first priority is to feel safe and take care of yourself.

While the chapters follow a sequence, it is absolutely fine to skip a practice or let a practice go—to return to later if you wish, or conclude it is not for you. You will still benefit from the other practices. This approach to healing is not a linear process.

Thich Nhat Hanh found that focused seated meditation was not always the most effective method of bringing mindfulness when his mind was very agitated, and thus he taught the practice of walking meditation and many other ways of applying mindfulness to daily life. We can take his guidance and try walking instead of sitting, with many of the meditations in this book.

Being a Soul Mate to Ourselves

In Vietnamese families, by tradition people do not usually say they love each other, believing that actions should speak louder than words. As a result, I cannot remember that my grandmother or my mother ever told me that they loved me. Still, the need to be told "I love you" was alive in me throughout my life, and I constantly searched for it in acknowledgment, attention, and affection from friends and boyfriends.

In my monastic life one day, while I was learning some Chinese characters, I discovered that the characters for "soul mate" literally mean "to remember, to know, and to master oneself"! This has been one of my most propitious enlightenments: directing my acknowledgment, attention, and affection toward myself and not waiting for or expecting anyone else to tell me I am loved. I have learned to tell myself "I love you" numerous times a day.

Self-love, to me, is every moment that we are mindful of our body, of our thoughts, of our feelings, breathing with what is arising without grasping or aversion. It is self-acceptance in practice. In fact, every moment that we are mindful of ourselves and of what is going on in us, we are meeting with ourselves as a soul mate. Every mindfulness practice discussed in this book enables us to realize this unconditional self-love.

Practice: Make a Time and Place for Healing

Whether or not we have sympathetic supporters for our healing, we always have ourselves. We can be our own soul mate.

Choose a place and time to be with yourself and reflect on healing for just fifteen minutes daily. Meditation instruction will come later, but for now, just think of finding time in your day. Sometimes it is helpful to reserve time for reflection at the beginning or the end of each day, on waking or when going to bed. Think of it as an appointment with your soul mate.

You may like to sit up to reflect in a special place, like in front of an altar; or you may like to lie down and relax; you may like to stand under a tree, or as I mentioned earlier, to take a regular walk outdoors. In a retreat in the Plum Village tradition, we create time for meditation in all four of these postures: sitting meditation, deep relaxation, standing meditation, and walking meditation. Think about how you would like to practice.

Find a notebook to write in and keep it by your bedside or on your desk, or if writing is difficult, you might find an app on your phone in which you can record your voice, which then transcribes your words for you to read at a later date. Your writing may take place as a journal, a poem, or a story, whichever form is most fluid for you at the moment.

Bringing poetry and music into your practice can infuse your being with joy, lightness, and mindfulness. Let yourself create freely without the need for form or appraisal. This is time for yourself.

Set an intention for healing during this special time in your day, when you will practice self-love and self-reflection.

Identify who in your family or circle of friends may be safe to share with in a one-on-one conversation. If there is no one with whom you feel safe, don't feel alone. Many survivors are in this position. This is just an indication that you may need to look outside of your current community for support and companionship on the path. In this case, consider joining a group dedicated to healing from trauma. Your *Sangha*—the Buddhist word for spiritual community—is also a wonderful source of support. The collective energy of practitioners can help us gradually feel safe in ourselves and in the presence of others. This is essential to our healing. See the Selected Resources section on page 262 to find a group or Sangha.

Sharing Our Experience

Recording, sharing, and writing about our experience is an invaluable tool for reflection. When we acknowledge what's going on and we write it down, the act of recording in itself can be therapeutic, helping us get our troubles "off our chest" so that they can then be seen and understood. Since ordaining as a nun, I myself have kept a journal on and off for many years.

When it comes to sharing with others, we may have trusted family members or friends, or we may have a relationship with a counselor or therapist whom we trust, who can help guide us and reflect our process back to us. However, many people with trauma do not have understanding friends or access to therapy. We may bravely try to share our experience with those around us, but find our suffering compounded rather than relieved.

I caution those of us who, driven by the need to share, may share indiscriminately—because some of our listeners may not be able to be empathetic at that moment, to listen to us or understand us, much less help us. If that is the case, we may put ourselves out there in a vulnerable position, while also watering the seed of suffering in us; we may force ourselves to relive our abuse, and suffer in so doing. We may retraumatize ourselves. Therefore, it is essential to remember why we share: it is for the sake of our own healing. We need to be aware of our surroundings and of the holding capacity in the people we entrust with our stories.

There tends to be two extremes when it comes to talking unskillfully about trauma. One is that we completely don't talk about it, don't write about it, and don't acknowledge it, even to ourselves. It's a way of trying to not allow it to exist; if we deny the existence of our trauma, we control it, or so we think. The other extreme is that sometimes we share about it a lot, write about it a lot, to the point that we may notice that we are neglecting other aspects of our lives. We become self-identified with our trauma and relate everything to it. We must question our own intention at these times and watch our own energy.

Denying and suppressing our suffering is unhealthy, but the other end of the spectrum, if we are not aware, can become a way of watering the seeds of suffering. Choose your listeners wisely, because the quality of their attention will affect your experience.

Sharing one's story with another person is a sacred experience and requires a correspondingly respectful listening ear; in the Plum Village monasteries, speaking from the heart and nonjudgmental deep listening have become a core part of our mindfulness practice.* However painful it may be, such sharing can become our teacher, helping us to deepen our humanity, our love, our understanding for ourselves and others. So we share with respect, in a space that is safe and healing for both the speaker (the person who shares) and the listener(s). It is important to hold the subject with respect and appropriateness.

So, when I share about sexual abuse, I don't share with just anybody. Now, as a monastic practitioner and a Dharma teacher, I share when I feel that my experience or insight can benefit others. Now I share not out of the need to heal myself—but because I know the practices that helped me to hold whatever I'm speaking about, and to heal it. I speak to help others through this journey, to make it easier for them and to encourage them to feel hopeful. My intention is to help make this happen for other people, because it's totally possible to heal on the spiritual journey if we receive good guidance and concrete practices.

Hungry Ghosts

In Buddhist traditions, we use the image of the hungry ghost to describe beings who are condemned to wander in a hell realm, unable to satisfy

---

* See chapter 11, "Loving Speech and Deep Listening" on page 221 for more about this mindfulness practice.

their emotional needs. Have you ever seen a drawing of a hungry ghost? Or have you perhaps seen a hungry ghost in real life? We have many hungry ghosts walking around in our society. A hungry ghost is a being with a throat that is needle-thin and a belly that is gravely extended. There is a feast in front of the hungry ghost, but because of its narrow neck, it cannot take in any nourishment. It also keeps everything inside, all bottled up.

Early in my monastic life, I recognized myself as a hungry ghost. Sometimes when I found it difficult to breathe because of strong emotions rising in me, I would put my hand on my throat and breathe, visualizing my throat gradually opening. I'd tell myself, "Just breathe, it's okay, I love you. Everything is okay, I'm still here." These simple statements have become my cherished mantras, effectively calming my nervous system and helping me to be kinder to myself and feel safe in my mind and body.

❀ *Practice: Self-Love and Loving Kindness*

If you are finding it hard to feel love for yourself, try the following short embodiment practices. Even if you don't have difficulties with self-love, it never hurts to take a moment to practice loving kindness toward yourself. You can do this anytime—at your workplace, in the car about to go somewhere, or as part of your daily mindfulness practice.

- Put one hand on your throat and breathe. Put another hand on your heart or on your belly and embrace yourself. Breathe gently, feeling the touch of your warm hand on the skin of your throat, for several in-breaths and out-breaths. If you feel safe, try gently closing your eyes.

- Tell yourself, "Just breathe. It's okay. I love you." Repeat as many times as you like.
- If it is difficult or uncomfortable to say, "I love you" to yourself at first, you can say, "Help me to love you. Help me to take better care of you."
- Move your hands to your opposite elbows and give yourself a hug. Feel the touch of your palms on your elbows. Hug yourself a little tighter, and then release. Do you feel the warmth and the life force in your own body? That is love right there.

How often do we acknowledge that, despite all the suffering that we might have gone through and put others through, life is still a feast to be enjoyed? There is a lot of love within us and all around us, as the energy of life.

- Try going outside for a walk, somewhere with trees and growing plants around you. Go with a friend, or go by yourself. Focus on soaking up the oxygen breathed out by the plants around you. Allow yourself to relax and touch love in the air, in the steps that you make, in the communal energy of living things. Do you feel love in the sunlight? Love is there, if only you would give yourself permission to taste it bit by bit.

There is a lot of love in our body. Our body is so faithful, so forgiving. We may have starved our body or stuffed it with food and relentless experiences; we may have deprived our body of sleep, of rest, of care, but our body continues to be there for us. It tries to heal again and again. Realizing my body's patience and resiliency, I have learned to come back to the breath, to the body, throughout the day, and to send a lot of love and gratitude to this body.

Sometimes we think negatively of our body, "You are ugly, you're not as beautiful as you should be, you're not as good as somebody else is...." Or we send a message to our body like, "I just want to die. Why aren't you dead?" Can you imagine what kind of energy that is? It is harsh, it's cruel, and it's powerful to send that sort of energy to ourselves. I have done that so many times in my life, and it becomes a habit. You just think of it, and many times you do not mean it. The self-hating thought rises up automatically, but it has the same effect whether you mean it or not. Your body still cringes. A dose of adrenaline is still released in your bloodstream. A sadness still sweeps through your body.

I had sent many harsh messages to my body, year after year. Eventually, my body got tired, and an insight came to me: it was like a boxer in a long match—you punch him, he falls, he gets up. You punch him again, he falls again, then he gets up. But if you keep punching him, at some point he's not going to be able to get back up. It's the same for ourselves. We are punishing ourselves if we keep sending ourselves unkind, unloving, cruel messages. "You're stupid. You're worthless. You're nobody. Go away! Just disappear!"

With the awareness we gain by practicing mindfulness and leading a spiritual life, we learn to recognize these messages, which I think of as "death wishes." Death wishes and self-loathing stem from unresolved traumas in our life, reflecting and feeding on one another. Therefore, we set an intention to protect ourselves first and foremost from our own injurious thoughts, speech, and behaviors, embracing ourselves and saying, "I'm sorry, I'm sorry, I don't mean that. Please help me to take better care of you." We can say to ourselves, "I am sorry that I never thought I was worthy of love."

In chapter 8, "Reverence for Life," we'll look more closely at suicidal thoughts and also offer ourselves the counterweight to this deep suffering: to hold deep respect for life, including our own life.* I have learned to tell myself, every time a death wish arises, "I don't have to wish for death. Death is taking place every moment. Every cell of my body goes through birth and death—some old cells die; some new cells are regenerated. It's a normal process."

Can I learn to live beautifully? Can I learn to heal my sadness and pain—for myself; for my partner who died; for my mother; for my father; for my brother; for Sunee, my young niece? Can I learn to heal myself for many? Can I learn to die beautifully every moment?

The answer to all these questions is yes. Let these thoughts and feelings of self-blame and self-hatred go. Breathe and release them as soon as they arise. Smile to them. That is learning to live beautifully and die beautifully.

Mindfulness Meditation

As Buddhist nuns, the most central practice we have in the monastery is to sit in mindfulness meditation, which can be a most relaxing and nourishing experience. Also, as we go about our daily life, if we can come back to our mindful breathing more often, the mind becomes much calmer, because it is one with the breath and with the body. The mind is not so busy running around and generating all sorts of comparisons and contrasts, discriminations, and preferences, and we can learn to relax.

However, when starting a meditation practice, we may find that it is difficult to be still. For this reason, we also practice walking meditation and other forms of more active practice. In this and the following

---

* See pages 179–195.

chapters, I will share some simple breathing, sitting, and walking meditation practices that you may find helpful in unraveling the knots of your tension, so that the process of healing can affect deeper levels of your body and consciousness.

🌼 *Practice: Breathing Flowers with Our Hands*

This is a simple practice to check in on your state of mind. Sit comfortably and rest your right or left hand on your lap or the arm of your chair. As you breathe in, close your hand gently. As you breathe out, open and relax your hand. You can start with one hand, then try with both hands, as your ability to maintain your awareness increases. Your hands are like flowers, opening and closing.

Breathing in, make a very gentle fist, but don't cause tension. Breathing out, just relax and let your hand open. See how many breaths you can follow and be aware of.

Most of us are hardly ever aware of our breathing. We rarely pay attention to it. Yet our breath is always available to us, wherever we are and whatever we are doing. While at work, sitting in class, or listening to someone's sharing, we can practice following what is happening along with our breathing.

This is a way of training our mind to stay with the body and thus to be more aware. However, don't give yourself a hard time if you find your mind wandering. The moment you notice that you've forgotten your breath is the moment you begin to be mindful again. Simply continue where you left off. Being kind and nonjudgmental with yourself is also a practice.

Developing your own practice is the center of your healing. There are many ways to obtain support, for example by finding a group of practitioners to sit with, in person or online. See the Selected Resources on page 262 to find a directory of practitioners. While connection to others is important, it is essential to first and foremost befriend yourself and your breathing as the foundation of your practice.*

🌸 *Practice: Following the Breath*

In my tradition, we compose short poems that we use in our mindfulness meditation, called *gathas*. These verses are similar to affirmations or statements to set intention, and I find them very helpful. The practice of following the breath will help increase the energy of awareness. You may like to find a place to sit quietly, with your spine straight but relaxed, and say the following verses in formal meditation. You can also say them to yourself throughout the day, to cultivate a sense of friendly support for yourself and your practice.

In guided meditation, a statement is given for the in-breath and another statement is given for the out-breath. Then they are followed by key words to help you focus your mind, so that you can continue to anchor your attention in your breathing as you practice looking deeply. The topic of this guided meditation is befriending our breathing. As you read each line of the poem, follow the breathing indicated by the words.

---

* The breathing exercises described here are rooted in the sixteen exercises of mindful breathing in the Buddha's Discourse on the Full Awareness of Breathing. The complete sixteen exercises are in the book by Thich Nhat Hanh, *Chanting from the Heart* (Berkeley, CA: Parallax Press, 2002). Thay's book *The Blooming of a Lotus* (Boston: Beacon Press, 2009) also offers many helpful guided meditation exercises.

Breathing in, I befriend my in-breath. [Inhale.]

Breathing out, I befriend my out-breath. [Exhale.]

In-breath [Inhale.]

Out-breath [Exhale.]

Breathing in, I simply observe the characteristics of my in-breath.
[Inhale.]

Breathing out, I simply observe the characteristics of my out-breath.
[Exhale.]

Observing in-breath [Inhale.]

Observing out-breath [Exhale.]

Breathing in, I follow my in-breath from the beginning to the end.
[Inhale.]

Breathing out, I follow my out-breath from the beginning to the end.
[Exhale.]

Following in-breath [Inhale.]

Following out-breath [Exhale.]

By observing and following our breathing in this way, we become conscious of the sensations of our breath in our body: the touch of air moving through our nostrils and the rise and fall of our chest and our abdomen. Gradually, we can bring our attention to all aspects of our being: our body, our steps, our actions, and gradually to our feelings of pain, fear, anxiety, and sadness as well. We gain an awareness of ourselves and loosen our strong sense of identification with the changing phenomena of our experience. Knowing how to take care of ourselves first, we then can go on to develop the capacity to recognize our suffering that is more deeply hidden.

Meditating while Walking

You can't really go wrong with walking meditation. In a retreat for teenagers at Deer Park Monastery, I asked one young man from Mississippi to give instructions on walking meditation to his peers. Standing in the middle of the circle, he started out with full confidence, saying, "Okay, take one step and breathe three, four times, and then take another step and breathe three, four times." Some teens started chuckling. "What?" he asked, hesitant and confused. "Or ... is it the other way around?"

 Practice: Basic Instructions for Walking Meditation

In walking meditation, you train to be aware of your breath and your steps simultaneously. By synching your breath to your steps, you cultivate the energy of mindfulness in your walking. At first you may feel awkward and unsteady in your steps, the way a beginner feels learning to dance. So, you incorporate one movement at a time, paying attention to the breath first, then to the steps, and then slowly incorporating the breath and the steps together.

Go slowly at first.

- Breathing in, take one, two, three steps.
- Breathing out, take two, three, four steps.

As you walk, you may like to quietly say an affirmation to yourself. I like to say, "Each step is peace," "Each step is healing," "Each step is love," and "Come back, come back to this moment."

In your daily life, the practice of walking meditation, from your bed to the bathroom, from your car to the office, everywhere you walk—*left foot, right foot, left foot, right foot, come back to the breath, come back to the breath*—enables you to live your life in that moment instead of being swept away by thoughts about the past, the future, or the present. What's going on may still sweep us away. But there is an island within you to come back to, and that is your mindful breathing and mindful steps.

Creating Safety by Listening

Since the time we were newborn infants, we began the quest for safety, expecting others to help us feel safe. We listened to our mother's cooing sound and to her calming voice. We looked to our parents and other caregivers for their pleasant facial expressions, supportive gestures, and loving embrace. As we grew older, our nervous system continued to assess other people's facial expressions, body movements, and vocal intonation as cues to determine whether or not they are safe people for us. Our senses and nervous systems perform this instant assessment and categorization automatically every time we meet a new person or situation, so we may not be consciously aware of it.

Because this behavior is involuntary, we may fall victim to a constant feeling of suspicion, fear, and a lack of safety, which cause us to react reflexively. The nervous system of survivors of trauma may be stuck in a state of hypervigilance, which may give rise to false alarms when there is actually no threat. We do not feel at ease with new people, a new environment, or a new situation.

It is extremely difficult for us to put down our guards and let others into our lives. Instead, we are constantly on the alert. I recognized this watchfulness in myself and in the teens I worked with in the San Francisco Youth Guidance Center, who had suffered from adverse childhood experiences. Among my medical school classmates, my friend Demond, who is Black, would immediately scan the place when walking into a room and locate the windows and the exit doors. While he had had a comfortable childhood, outside his home he did not feel safe in the United States as a Black man. It was sometimes difficult for me to connect with him because he would constantly look around and be on alert at sudden sounds or the appearance of strangers. Even when we were having dinner in a nice restaurant, Demond still behaved this way. One time, seeing the upset expression on my face, Demond muttered, "Sorry. It's a habit."

When we have undergone traumatic violence, we may constantly look behind ourselves, and even a hug or a tap on the shoulder from behind can give us a fright. We might prefer to sit facing the door and with our backs against the wall, so that if anything were to happen, we could run out the door or jump out of the window quickly. On the whole, we tend to not like surprises and may prefer to gather in small circles of friends, going through life avoiding environments that trigger us.

How can we begin to undo the lifelong habit of being on high alert? The practice of deep listening to the breath and body can help us assess situations with more awareness and accuracy. We begin to move away from involuntary, habitual behaviors. We can proactively create feelings of safety and calm in ourselves and in the presence of others, so that we can develop meaningful relationships. Practicing mindfulness with our spiritual community is optimal for this purpose. All our practices—sitting meditation, walking meditation, eating meditation, singing practice songs, deep relaxation, listening to Dharma talks and Dharma sharing—generate the collective energy of safety, peace, and calmness.

Hospital Environments

One night when I was doing a rotation in the emergency room at UCSF General Hospital, a rape victim was brought in for examination whom I will never forget. I walked by the room and saw her curled up in a chair, all alone, waiting to be seen by a doctor. The lighting in the exam room was too bright. Everything looked too cold and sterile. Her body looked small and vulnerable. I felt so sorry for a girl so young, so alone in that environment. It was the opposite of a soft place to land. I wanted to go in to talk to her and offer her some comfort, but I had my own patients to tend to, and it was a busy night. Each time I walked by the room, I looked at her, still curled up all alone for hours.

Twenty-plus years have passed, and the sight of her is still with me, together with a gnawing feeling of regret for not having reached out to comfort her, even for just a few minutes. How frightening and lonesome it must have been for her to be in that exam room, without parents or friends or even doctors or nurses to express some sort of warm feeling toward her! That lonesome experience in the exam room was traumatic, and it must have compounded her rape trauma further.

However traumatic a situation may be, if we who are present in the immediate aftermath—the medical professionals, family members, friends, social workers, the police, the hospital staff—can act as a supportive community for the traumatized individual and help take care of the person as mindfully, kindly, and peacefully as we can, this empathy and thoughtfulness will ameliorate the severity of their situation. Then with further time and space to rest, to process, to reflect, and to understand the experience, true healing can take place and when we recall the experience in the future, we will remember others' warmth and humanity instead of further trauma. That is why taking care of the healing process is so important.

Recently, I received a letter from Laura, a high-school student I had been mentoring for a while. She recounted the story of her recent admission to a psychiatric hospital, and it immediately reminded me of what I had witnessed in the ER twenty-odd years ago. It confirmed for me that many hospitals in the United States are still struggling to provide a truly healing environment for patients.

My sister called the police to take me to the hospital. This was the third time I had been forced to go to the hospital because of my suicidal thoughts. I was so scared the whole time, nervous and anxious. There were many policemen standing inside my apartment, not allowing me to touch even my personal stuff. I had to go straight to the hospital with them, wearing my pajamas.

Sitting in the back of the police car, handcuffed, I was overwhelmed by humiliation. It brought me back to one of my past traumas. I cried a lot on the way to the hospital.

"Why do I have no freedom to decide my own life?"

"When will I have a control of my life?"

"Why did I end up being at the same place again?"

Thousands of "whys" whirled inside my head, nearly exploding my mind.

In the first hospital, I still had some good luck because I met some nice staff, including a nurse, a nurses' aide, a therapist, and a guard. They took good care of me and asked me why I came there.... After I calmed down and breathed for a while, they lent me a computer to do my homework and I journaled to give myself some encouragement and to express my painful emotions. The nurse praised me for being productive, and she brought me snacks and water. I was smiling brightly, so she told me, "You look so happy, not like other patients. I cannot understand why you are in here. But anyways, keep smiling bright like that and keep studying to become a scientist. I don't want to see you in here again." I smiled and thanked her.

After the doctor saw me, he thought that I should switch my prescription from bupropion to lithium, so he transferred me to the psychiatric hospital to recheck my medicine and my condition before I could go home.

The psychiatric hospital was truly terrifying! Just being there was traumatizing, and I could not see how it was in any way healing or helping any of the people who were unlucky enough to be admitted there long-term. The therapists there were overwhelmed, emotionless, and numb to the patients. Even though I was there only overnight and discharged the next morning, what I saw continues to haunt me until now. The rooms were cold and the indifferent treatment toward patients reminded me of those movies about prison. The guards were huge, always following and watching the patients closely. A nurse told me that if I had any questions, I could ask the therapists and nurses, but they were always on their computers at the nursing station. Some patients were wandering the corridors, some were screaming, and some were sleeping all the time. The atmosphere was heavy and tense.

This hospital didn't allow the patients to keep their phones or laptops, and even my treasured necklace with the pendant of the Bodhisattva of Deep Listening was confiscated. We were treated like crazy prisoners, and it was very disempowering. I couldn't eat anything that night. Instead, I asked for a few pages of paper and colored pencils to draw.

I was so scared, and I cried a lot. But then slowly I calmed myself down and comforted myself that I was only there for just one night, waiting for the doctor to check my medication. Instead of paying attention to my chaotic surroundings, I began to practice walking meditation, focusing on my breath and steps in order to calm my anxiety. After a while, I felt better. My terror and other emotions calmed down.

As Laura's story shows, a patient's experience in the hospital can determine the direction of their healing process, and suffice it to say, patients going through trauma are all too often retraumatized by the hospital itself! Hospital leaders and administrators need to do more to make these places more welcoming and healing for the patients, and provide something technology and medication can never offer: empathy and human understanding.

There are few things that can make a person feel more safe, heard, and protected than the presence of a good listener. If we did not have anyone to listen to us after a traumatic experience, like Laura, we can create for ourselves an atmosphere of safety by being a soul mate to ourselves here and now.

❀ *Practice: Listening to Your Breath and Body*

A soul mate is someone who can listen to you with equanimity. In fact, this is what you do in sitting meditation: you listen to yourself, being your own soul mate and providing yourself with a feeling of safety and security. This same capacity will enable you to listen to the thoughts and feelings of others, too. Find a quiet and safe distraction-free place to practice deep listening to your own breath and body.

LISTENING TO YOUR BREATH

Breathing in, I listen to my in-breath.

Breathing out, I listen to my out-breath.

In-breath, out-breath

Listening, smiling

*[You can quietly repeat these key words in italics to help you culti-
vate your mindfulness and concentration.]*

Breathing in, I am aware that my in-breath is telling me that it
is short, rapid, and loud (or it is long, slow, and quiet).

Breathing out, I am aware that my out-breath is telling me that
it is ...

Aware of what the breath is telling me

Breathing and relaxing

LISTENING TO YOUR BODY

Breathing in, I listen to my body.

Breathing out, I listen to my body.

Listening to my body

I'm here for you!

Breathing in, I am aware that my body is telling me that it is tired,
tense, and restless (or it is relaxed, calm, and at ease, etc.).

Breathing out, I am aware that my body is telling me that it is ...

Aware of what my body is telling me

I listen. I listen.

Variation: Listening to Another Person's Breath

When you are a soul mate to yourself, you will be able to be a soul mate to another person, anchoring in your own breath and body while being aware of that person's breath and body.

1. Establish yourself in the awareness of your own breath.
2. Establish yourself in the awareness of your own breath and body.
3. Listen to the other person's breath. What insight do you gain?

> Breathing in, I listen to the in-breath of the person in front
> of me.
> Breathing out, I listen to their out-breath.
> *In-breath, out-breath*
> *Listening, smiling*

Once you become more comfortable with this practice of listening to the breath and body of your own and of another person in a quiet and safe space, experiment and bring your practice to other situations where you are with more people and in a less controlled environment. Notice how this awareness may affect the quality of your being, your listening, and your sense of safety and comfort.

CHAPTER 2

The Way Out Is In

*When you breathe in, you bring your mind home to your body. A lot of
the time, your mind is not with your body. But when they are together, you
are truly in the here and the now for your transformation and healing.
It is wonderful to be present and your breath becomes the object of your
mind and you can become a free person. You can cultivate freedom.*

—THICH NHAT HANH

My teacher often said, "The way out is in." What did he mean by "the
way out"? He was referring to the exit from suffering, despair, jealousy,
anxiety, depression, superstition, and all the mental states that haunt
us day and night, giving us no rest. But what did he mean by going *in*?

First of all, "the way in" means to gather mindfulness, concentration, and insight into our own body and mind, or more specifically, into
what we call the five "aggregates" or *skandhas* of our being: our body,
feelings, mental formations, perceptions, and consciousness. Instead
of looking only at the outward causes of our suffering, we look inward.
When we learn to look inwardly at ourselves—with love, but also with
a degree of equanimity, to observe how our mental states derive from
a sense of our identity as a separate self—we can find a path out of
suffering.

Taking Care of Our Mind

As a doctor, I worked with many patients in their dying hours. They would scream or cry, drenched in despair. All their untended relationships and unresolved pain would surge and become uncontrollable. In their last moments, deep-seated complexes would manifest in their mind with no mercy.

To die peacefully, we need to live peacefully. But how? We need to take care of our mental formations while we still have time, long before the moment of death. In my book *Mindfulness as Medicine,* I shared a near-death experience I had when the brakes suddenly failed on a car I was driving at high speed. I came flying off the freeway with no way to slow down. It was the kind of exit ramp that spirals downward, and I knew I would not be able to stop. Holding on to the wheel, I saw my life like the frames of a movie flashing through my mind at the speed of light. I didn't think about it, and there was no time to use my intellectual understanding, I just saw-understood, saw-understood, saw-understood. I grasped exactly what each of those moments was about immediately, with no evaluation. At times like this, when we are close to death, our mind reveals our whole life to us in lightning flashes.

I kept steering and the car ran through red lights and green lights until it finally came to a stop on a deserted street. Overwhelmed, I immediately tumbled out of the driver's seat and walked and walked until I found a supermarket and went in to get help. Not until after I became a nun did I make time to reflect and gain valuable insights from this experience.

I came to see my unfinished business. I learned that the mind has a mechanism for trying to understand what is going on in our life and to resolve it. But if we are preoccupied with other matters—for example, if we are caught up in our work, or in the pursuit of fame, success, or satisfaction on a superficial level—then the deeper needs are not addressed. The mind continues to try to process our traumas in our waking life and especially in our dreams. If we do not address the deep-seated complexes, suppressing them or running away from them, then this rumination and regurgitation of the mind becomes a habit. We suffer, but have no way of embracing that suffering.

Unconscious habitual actions become our way of life and form the path that we inevitably and inadvertently travel down. So, we need to learn to take care of our unfinished business in our daily life, bit by bit, whether that is depression, anger, resentment, sadness, or other types of pain. As we address the past, we also take care of the present moment because the present moment soon becomes the past and serves as the foundation for the future. We have this one chance to live in the here and now and to transform and heal, so that we don't have to chase after the tail of the past. In fact, we can only resolve our unfinished business in the here and now.

The past is gone, and the future has not yet come. What we truly have control over is the present. Learn to breathe, relax, and have right view, a way of perceiving the world as it is, so that we may engage with life most appropriately; and the mind does not have to regurgitate and ruminate past suffering anymore.

Rehearsing Suffering

A major obstacle to meditation is the tendency of our mind to get stuck in negative thinking. The mind "rehearses" the scenarios that bother us, ultimately because it wants to resolve the problem and to find a way out. Unfortunately, it may get stuck in its track like the needle of the gramophone stuck in a groove, repeating the same track ceaselessly.

Trauma survivors are frequently troubled by repetitive intrusive thinking. The mind has been likened to a search engine—you initiate a thought and it gives you other thoughts related to it. For example, if we keep harboring hateful thoughts, they lead to more hate and violence. In the article "From Hate to Love: An Ex-Neo-Nazi's Journey to Buddhism," Arno Michaelis, a former white supremacist, shared that he had been ruthlessly violent to people of color. After his conversion to Buddhism, when asked how people could inflict pain on others and even murder them, he replied, "Practice. When you practice hate and violence, it makes your life so miserable that nothing but homicide followed by suicide seems to make sense. Things like love and compassion and forgiveness and kindness and all the most beautiful aspects of our human experience not only become unfamiliar but repulsive to you."[*]

Everything we routinely do can be understood as practicing and rehearsing. With this awareness, we learn to use our search engine mindfully and selectively put in our search bar only positive elements. In neuroscience, it is known that neurons that "fire together wire together."[**] When certain neurons fire together continuously, over time the connection becomes stronger between those neurons. The triggering factor may be a thought, a word or sentence, or an action, and then a particular neural pathway is immediately activated, via electrical impulses and then the release of neurotransmitters—a whole chain reaction takes place instantly, just as an often-used trail becomes a well-worn path.

---

[*]   Kyte, Lindsay, and Lion's Roar Staff. "An Ex-Neo-Nazi's Journey to Buddhism." *Lion's Roar*. May 16, 2018. Accessed October 16, 2020. https://www.lionsroar.com/an-ex-neo-nazis-journey-to-buddhism/.

[**]   "Hebbian Learning and Predictive Mirror Neurons for Actions, Sensations, and Emotions," Christjan Keysers and Valeria Gazzola, The National Center for Biotechnology Information, www.ncbi.nlm.nih.gov/pmc/articles/PMC4006178/.

Frequently activated neural pathways may begin to function automatically, manifesting as a habit or a habitual pattern—and this becomes your personality over time. Similarly, for people with PTSD, they only need to hear a sudden sound, see something triggering, or even just think of an unpleasant experience, and immediately a whole cascade of reactions, thoughts, speech, and behaviors ensues. Someone who has been abused may be repulsed by the touch of their lover, or a combat soldier may start to scream exactly as if they were in a war zone. In this way, the trauma doesn't happen only once; it happens physiologically every time we relive it traumatically with our thoughts. Even when you have a nightmare, your whole body goes through it—neurotransmitters are released.

When you do or say something negatively the first time, you may feel bad about it, but the second time it may already feel less unsettling. You may tell yourself "You're not worthy," or you may scream at your spouse, or hit the wall—the first time you do it, it is a shock. But the second time you may feel less bad. And then the behavior may become a habit. Every time you get angry, you punch the wall. It can become uncontrollable. A habit becomes a personality, which then determines the course of your life and destiny.

We have to rehearse in a positive way, so it gets easier to see the positive side of a situation. This relates to how we perceive our reality, which we discuss in more detail in this chapter. The sign or appearance of the object or situation may be exactly the same, but the state of mind determines how we perceive the situation. By practicing the Five Strengths, we can train our mind to be in a state of spaciousness: calm, positive, and able to perceive the situation with more clarity, equanimity, and a sense of possibility.

Of course, genetic predisposition is a factor. Some people have inherited positive mindsets from their families, seeing the sunny side of life more easily. Their families may have a strong culture of appreciation and respect for each other. If you are one of those fortunate people, you can always practice more to recognize the subtle thoughts of judgment, discrimination, and anger, so that you can be even happier and help uplift others.

For those of us who tend to be gloomy and in despair easily, compounded with the suffering of the past, our habitual mood makes it even more difficult to handle and transform the situation. Then we really need to have right view and right thinking. We train to be aware of what we are thinking and to breathe with it, relax it, and change it to a more balanced view, recognizing the good conditions that are still available to us. We can remind ourselves, "Smile. Choose to think of it in a positive way." The more we become aware of positive conditions, however minimal they are, the more grateful we become. The Five Strengths and the Five Mindfulness Trainings in parts 2 and 3 of this book provide active training in rehearsing for a joyful and content existence. It is entirely possible to create new, mindful, positive habits. This is certainly possible with the practice of loving speech and deep listening toward ourselves. Positivity and gratitude slowly become a new, mindful habit.

In my years as a novice nun, it was challenging for me to come back to the breath during sitting meditation. Morning or evening, I would sit down and fall asleep, nodding off before the bell master started the opening chant. I felt exhausted and feeble. While I was dozing, my mind went into dark and gloomy places, where indiscernible thoughts were lurking, muddled up in negative energy.

Perhaps sleepiness was one of the ways my hypervigilant mind was trying to protect me from my own harmful thoughts. Unwittingly, it created a vicious cycle since those murky thoughts begot further negativity and despair.

Our thoughts are often like that as we go about our daily lives unaware. We may even believe it's normal to *think* all the time, when we're awake or even when we're sleeping. But it's not normal, in fact. Thay called it "the nonstop radio of the mind." Indeed, it is life leakage, losing our life energy through every thought that is undetected and unrecognized. I'm not talking about creative thinking, or exercising the intellect, but about unconscious self-talk, driven by stress, fear, and anxiety. These thoughts in turn can lead to more thoughts, speech, and bodily actions that are self-destructive and hurtful to ourselves and others. Habituated to continually thinking, we may not know or remember what peace of mind is like anymore.

Another time, when I was seriously ill for three years with Lyme disease, I couldn't sit in meditation at all. However, I did my best to anchor my attention in my breath, so at least I did not get lost in a black hole of negative thoughts and sensations. Thanks to this practice of anchoring my mind in my breath, I saved my mind and, in fact, became more mindful of my breathing in daily life.

Our subconscious mind has all the seeds of different mental formations within it, both beneficial and harmful. The seeds to which we give attention grow and become strongly rooted, forming habits. That's why it is important to take care of our complexes and problems as soon as we become aware of them, while it is easiest to work with them.

Three Complexes

Due to our past experiences, we trauma survivors may encounter a major block to looking inward; we rarely experience enough psychological safety to stop and look into the content of our mind. While we may be able to function quite well in our daily lives, we may be in a chronic state of hypervigilant stress.

The human mind constantly assigns value and classification to experience as part of its survival mechanism, aiming for safety as its crucial goal. As a result, we spend our lives looking outward, in a state of vigilance, to avoid being harmed or traumatized again. We think of ourselves as people to whom bad things will happen, and strive to keep a sense of separation from others to avoid being hurt.

Three very powerful complexes arise together with the sense of a separate self: inferiority, superiority, and equality complexes. We may find ourselves expending energy running between extremes of trying to prove our worth, or beating ourselves up for our unworthiness. We may think "I'm better than you," or "I'm just as good as you," or "Gosh, I'm not as good, I'm not good enough." In so-called "normal" culture, in which competition is frequently valued over cooperation, our whole society joins in creating and reinforcing these complexes.

Even if we don't feel physically threatened in our bodies, we may transfer our sense of self to our achievements and possessions, and compare ourselves to others via our education, our jobs, the cars we drive, or the size of our homes or bank accounts. We constantly struggle with these complexes and assign value to our experience. We put ourselves up for auction, tormented with the question, "How much am I worth?"

If we don't practice to identify these complexes in us, we may lose touch with our inherent sense of worth. Sadly, it doesn't matter how successful, how accomplished, how rich, how powerful, how senior in society we may become; we still act so insecure, because we are trapped in this notion of a separate, defensive self. We are always trying to compete, to compare ourselves with others and try to outdo them. We may even be competitive about our trauma and our healing practices.

We're always coming up with some scheme to protect ourselves, to protect the "me" and the "my." The antidote to the three complexes is unconditional self-love and self-acceptance. Please follow the self-love practices in the previous chapter on pages 20–21. Meditation is an invitation to let go of these complexes, to stop judging and comparing ourselves with others, and to lay down the armor of a separate self, so we can experience real safety and spaciousness of mind.

Perceptions and Our State of Mind

The body is the most concrete form of ourselves that we can be aware of. Then we have the mind that manifests our feelings, which can be pleasant, unpleasant, neutral, or mixed. We also have mental formations or states of mind, which include perceptions about each other and ourselves. While these perceptions can determine our happiness and our suffering, we actually know very little about them. My teacher, Thich Nhat Hanh, has said that 99 percent of our perceptions are incorrect!

The Chinese character for "perception" or "to perceive" is 想. The upper half of the character is composed of the root characters for "tree" and "eye," which together represent "sign" or "appearance." The eye sees the tree, and it recognizes it. The lower half is the root character for "mind" or "heart."

When "sign" and "mind" come in contact, perception arises. This character 想 "to perceive," when used in conjunction with other characters in different contexts, can also mean "to assume," "to imagine," "to anticipate," "to project into the future," or "to reminisce."

Thus, the composition of the character tells us that it's the state of the mind and its previous experiences that determine what a person actually "sees." For example, the "sign" may be a tree, but when the mind is involved, the perception may become "that's a beautiful tree" or even "that's a dangerous tree"—if, for example, the person had been struck by a similar falling tree before. The Chinese character 想 reflects that there is not one fixed reality and helps explain why it is important to understand our mind. The mind determines how we may view ourselves and the world in a distorted way, especially because of past trauma and negative experiences.

We find the way out of suffering and ill-being by looking deeply into the working of our mind and how it may view our five skandhas of body, feelings, mental formations, perceptions, and consciousness. When we have a clear understanding about who we are, we learn to take care of ourselves appropriately in each present moment, where life truly exists. Moreover, we can train our mind to be in a state of spaciousness, calm and positive, so as to perceive the situation with more clarity, equanimity, and a sense of possibility.

❁ *Practice: You Think So?*

Upon my request, Thay once wrote me a calligraphy that said "You think so?" Asking this question is a great practice to check in with our perceptions. It helps us reexamine our deeply ingrained views and perceptions, so that we may discover ourselves from different angles and at deeper levels.

In my spiritual life, I have found myself having to yield and release layer after layer of views, perceptions, and attitudes that I once thought were solid and immovable. Letting go of fixed opinions has allowed me to accept myself and be accepted by others; to experience joy, and to be okay with it, and not cling to my suffering.

Practicing self-inquiry with the question, "You think so?" has taught me so much about how I think about suffering. "It's mine! You don't understand it. My pain is greater than your pain." It takes a lot of courage to release and let go of our negativity.

Let's try this practice. For example, say you have a negative thought toward yourself, such as "That's awful!" or "That was really dumb what I said." Breathe, smile, and ask yourself, "You think so?"

Continue to breathe, smile, and listen for a while.

Has anything changed?

You think so?

Reflection: The Mindful Horse

Being able to stop the habit of incessant thinking is a great power. I'm sure you have been in situations when you don't want to think certain thoughts anymore, but you keep thinking them. Or, you know certain actions or words may damage your relationships further, but you can't stop yourself from continuing to do or say harmful things.

To be able to stop is something we can cultivate in our daily life: to let go, come back to our breath, and release the negative thought with an out-breath. Release that gesture, just relax the body with the out-breath. And so daily, we train in ourselves a capacity to release, to let go and relax that tension in the body and in the perception.

Imagine an improbable scenario: riding on a horse that is galloping wildly through an art and history museum filled with many beautiful interesting objects. Yet this is what our situation is like. We would not be able to see much or enjoy the exhibits. However, the moment you slow down, stop, and get off from the horse and calm him down enough to stand still, you may see the exquisite intricacies of the artwork that you previously missed. That is mindfulness.

The mind is like that horse. To be able to quiet the mind, to see and to know what's going on inside and all around, right here and right now: that is mindfulness. To rein in the mind, we use mindful breathing as a rope to hold the horse, helping it to be calm. Mindful breathing is like an anchor for the mind.

Although we cannot see, hear, smell, taste, or touch the mind, we can definitely feel the breath with our five senses. On a winter day, we can see the moisture in our breath condensing in the cold air. We can hear our own breathing, whether it's gentle or coarse, slow or rapid. We can smell the breath. We can touch the breath and feel its temperature and moisture. So, with our five sense organs, and with the mind as our sixth sense, we can perceive and recognize the characteristics of our breathing.

Our breaths are physiological manifestations of our mind. When we are anxious, we breathe differently; when we are startled, we hold our breath; and when are angry, our breathing becomes faster and shallower. As we relax, our breathing becomes slower and deeper, and we can feel the rising and the falling of our abdomen. In fact, the Chinese character for "breath" is 息, which means "from the mind" or "the mind itself"!*

In these ways, our breathing patterns reflect our state of mind. Mindful breathing helps us to be more aware of the galloping of our habitual mind, slowing it down gradually to a stop. Mindful breathing starts with the awareness of our in-breaths and out-breaths. We explore our breathing by recognizing where we can feel the breath entering us: at the nose level, at the mouth level, at the chest level, or at the abdominal level.

---

* The root character 自 means "actual" or "originating from" and 心 means "mind" or "heart," together forming 息, the character "breath."

You may like to try to stop the horse of your thinking from time to time during the day, by pausing whatever you are doing. At the monastery where I live, we practice pausing with all different kinds of bells, such as the telephone rings, the activity bell, the church bell, etc. For example, whenever we hear the phone ring, we stop talking and moving about and remember to enjoy our breathing. Whenever the dining room clock chimes, we stop talking or eating and check in with our breathing and our feelings. In this way, even outside the meditation hall, we have ample opportunities to cultivate mindfulness and ease.*

Intelligence in the Body

In Buddhist psychology, there are pleasant feelings, unpleasant feelings, mixed feelings, and neutral feelings. A feeling is a mental phenomenon, but it is experienced in the body. For example, we may feel our heart fluttering when we are happy, pounding or tightening when we are angry or anxious. Awareness of the body *in the body* helps us recognize feelings as they arise, allowing our intelligence to distinguish them and investigate their root cause. For example, sometimes we may have anxiety, but without self-awareness, we may mistake anxiety for hunger, so we turn to food for comfort. If we are not able to feel satisfied by the food we eat, it may be because we are numb to our body, so then we continue to eat, trying to fill a void that is bottomless, and becoming enchained in a vicious cycle of binging and self-loathing. Awareness in this way brings about a deeper understanding of the feelings and vice versa, enabling us to break through this vicious cycle.

We used to believe that the brain constantly sends orders to the heart, the digestive system, and the rest of the body. Within the last

---

* See the Selected Resources on page 262 for a simple mindfulness bell recommendation.

twenty years, research has found that the heart sends more signals to the brain than the brain to the heart, and not the other way around, thus prompting the coining of the term "heart brain."[*] This is also true for the digestive tract, which also sends more signals to the brain than the brain to the guts: we now recognize we have a "gut brain." In this vein, we can talk about our "lung brain" or even our "skin brain." Our whole body is alive and intelligent, constantly sending signals to the head brain. More than 2,600 years ago, Indian yogis as well as the Buddha must already have had this enlightenment about the interbeing nature of these centers of intelligence and their two-way communication when they developed their meditative practices.

Signals from the body, including the "heart brain" and "gut brain," have a significant effect on the "head brain," influencing emotional processing as well as higher cognitive faculties such as attention, perception, memory, and problem-solving. All parts of our body constantly send messages to each other, listen to each other, respond to each other, and give feedback. There is no one "boss" in the individual organs.

We can apply this knowledge to take better care of ourselves and our trauma. Instead of paying exclusive attention to only our "head brain" and getting lost in thoughts, perceptions, memories, and feelings that may be abstract, vague, and overwhelming, the practice of "awareness of the body in the body" helps us to tune in to the more concrete and accurate messages sent to us from the lungs, the heart, the gut, and the body as a whole. This practice helps us gain better understanding and insight into the present state of our body and mind. It also facilitates and reintegrates our head brain–body brain connection, so that there is more harmony and coherence. This practice can be particularly

---

* Dr. J. Andrew Armour. "Chapter 01: Heart-Brain Communication." HeartMath Institute. Accessed October 17, 2020. https://www.heartmath.org/research/science-of-the-heart/heart-brain-communication/.

healing for survivors of trauma who have PTSD symptoms or feel dis-embodied or alienated from the body.

Like all our animal ancestors, humans are on a perennial quest for safety. When our own physiological states are in balance, we feel set-tled, calm, and safe. Only then can restoration, growth, and healing take place; only then can we can be open to ourselves and others on a more intimate level. Therefore, it is essential to be aware of the messages sent from our body, specifically from our heart brain, our lung brain, and our guts brain. These messages are both physiological and emotional. The practice of simple recognition of these messages and breathing and relaxing with them can calm and soothe our nervous system at all levels, which gives us a feeling of safety and ease. This is particularly important to survivors of trauma because our body is constantly revved up, causing us to often feel jittery, apprehensive, and unsafe.

Stay with any one exercise for as long as you need before you move on to the next exercise.

❊ *Practice: Listening to Our Lung Brain*

In this exercise, you listen to the physiological messages specifically coming from your lungs, including your respiratory rate, the quality of your breathing, any chest wall pain or tightness, or any sensations aris-ing from your chest area. You can quietly repeat the key words in italics at the end of each verse to aid your concentration and meditation.

Sit or lie somewhere quiet. Tune in to listen to the sensations and emotional messages that are issued from your "lung brain," such as a feeling of ease versus suffocation; expansiveness versus tightness or withdrawal; or lightness and happiness versus feeling heavy and crushed, and so on. Smile, rest, and release any pain or tension in your chest in every pause between the in-breaths and the out-breaths.

> Breathing in, I become aware of my breath.
> Breathing out, I listen to my breath.
> *Aware of breathing, listening.*
> *Thank you! Thank you!*

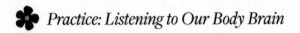 Practice: Listening to Our Body Brain

In this exercise, you listen to the general messages of your body, such as whether it is relaxed or tense or jittery; comfortable or in pain; upright and open, or slouched and drawn in. Listen also to the messages sent from the skin, muscles, and joints.

Then you can tune in to the sensations and emotional messages from your body brain, such as a feeling of ease versus tension; stability versus irritability or restlessness; or lightness and happiness versus heavy, sad feelings in the body.

As you scan through your body and the feelings in your body, stay anchored in your in-breaths and out-breaths, relaxing the physical as well as the emotional body with your mindful breathing and relaxation. Smile, rest, and release any pain or tension in every pause between the in-breaths and the out-breaths.

> Breathing in, I become aware of my body brain.
> Breathing out, I listen to the message of my body by scanning
>   through my body from head to toe.
> *Aware of body, listening, relaxing*
> *I listen. I listen.*

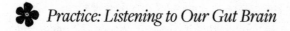 Practice: Listening to Our Heart Brain

Messages from the heart may manifest in the form of lightness or heaviness of the chest; relaxing or tightening, crushing pain in the chest; pleasant, slow, regular, or rapid, irregular heartbeats, and so on. In this exercise, you listen to the rate and rhythm of the heart from inside your body. It may help to place your hand on the very center of your chest, over your heart.

Listen deeply to the sensations and emotional messages that are reflected from your heart brain, such as feelings of peace, joy, openness, gratitude, or melancholy, sadness, fury, pain.

Remember to stay anchored in your breathing and in your body, relaxing the physical as well as the emotional heart with your mindful breathing and relaxation. Smile, rest, and release the tension and pain in every pause between the in-breaths and the out-breaths.

> Breathing in, I listen to my heart brain.
> Breathing out, I become aware of the message sent from my
>   heart brain.
> *Aware of heart brain, listening*
> *I am here for you.*

Practice: Listening to Our Gut Brain

Messages from the gut at the first level may include the rise and fall of the abdomen; the distention or tightness of the abdomen; rumbling sounds from the intestines; lightness or queasiness; dull pain or discomfort; or knotted, "butterfly" sensations in the stomach.

Listen to the deeper sensations and emotional messages that are reflected from your gut brain. They may be feelings of safety, ease, and settlement, or unsettlement, insecurity, worry, excitement, or fear.

Continue to stay anchored in your breathing and in your body, relaxing the physical as well as the emotional feeling of your abdominal area with your mindful breathing and relaxation. Smile, rest, and release any tension and pain in every pause between the in-breaths and the out-breaths.

Congratulations! As you are practicing these exercises, you are being a soul mate to yourself, present to remember, to know, and to care for what is in your body and mind.

Every single practice that we follow in our monasteries—from mindful breathing and sitting meditation, to mindful walking, mindful eating, mindful working, mindful speaking and listening, to deep relaxation—is to train our mind to stop running away to the past and to the future. In other words, we stop the runaway horse of our unconscious habitual actions. You may argue that these practices work only in the calm surroundings of a monastery, which is unlike the busy life you live out here. In fact, these practices work well even when you live a busy life in surroundings that look nothing like the serenity of a monastery. When we do our practices with the qualities of the Five Strengths, as offered in the next part of this book, we will benefit from them at the deepest levels of the mind and body. Our practices serve as a special training for our wild mind so that it becomes cooperative and loving, allowing us to enjoy our life journey with a deeper sense of purpose and ease. They help the mind to dwell in the here and now, so that we can live our lives freely and touch deep happiness.

PART 2

THE *five* STRENGTHS

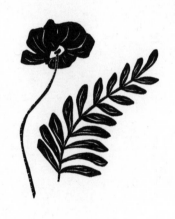

CHAPTER 3

Trust as a Strength

When you love someone, you have to have trust and confidence. Love without trust is not yet love. Of course, first you have to have trust, respect, and confidence in yourself.

—THICH NHAT HANH

Claire came to our monastery for retreats when she was in her teens. She confided in me that when she was a child, her maternal grandparents would babysit regularly, and her grandfather would get her alone and sexually molest her. Her grandmother never seemed to notice. Even her parents failed to pay attention to the fact that their child was disheveled and distraught, at times crying when they picked her up. One time she came running to the front door naked, yet the parents did not investigate.

According to Claire, when she finally told her mother, her mother scolded her and said she was making it up. Claire thought her mother was in denial and could not believe that her father could do such a thing to his granddaughter. Claire had been wronged, and then she was accused of lying. These wounds severely affected Claire's teenage years and eventually severed her relationship with her grandparents and her parents.

Years later, after Claire had become an adult, I finally met her mother, Johanna. An advocate for young people, Johanna worked to prevent the abuse of children. She had heard Claire talking about me, and she came to me for help and insight into the reasons for her daughter's cutting off ties with her family. Johanna sincerely wanted to know if something had happened to her daughter in childhood, because, she observed, Claire's personality and her relationship with everyone in the family had completely changed. Johanna could recall some signs of distress, but she was not sure if "something had been going on."

After asking her several questions to confirm her genuine intention, I told Johanna what had happened to Claire. She was heartbroken when I confirmed her father's abuse of her daughter. She revealed that she herself had been abused by a cousin in her childhood, and her entire professional career was dedicated to advocating for children and protecting them from sexual abuse. Yet she had failed to keep her own child out of harm's way. In Johanna's own memory, she had tried to coax Claire to tell her what was happening to her when she saw that her daughter was becoming distant and withdrawn, but the girl refused to say anything.

Here we can see how two people may have different recollections of the same event: Claire experienced her mother contradicting her and accusing her of lying, while Johanna recalled trying to find out what had happened but being met by obstinate silence. Mother and daughter were both suffering greatly. Most likely, as a child Claire had tried to communicate with her mother about the abuse in her own way and in her own language, but her mother had failed to understand her and remove her promptly from the harmful environment. Johanna, unable to see what was in front of her own eyes, had not responded to Claire's needs. The mother was carrying her own hidden internal pain from her own childhood, making it even harder for her to acknowledge Claire's situation.

Thus, Claire had lost trust in her mother and given up on further communication. The relationship between parent and child, instead of being a source of love, became a source of tension and division, a deep betrayal that destroyed Claire's trust in herself as well as in her family. If we look around in our communities, we may observe many families with similar broken relationships, in which contact is minimal or nonexistent, with fragile areas that cannot be discussed or brought to light. Our own family of origin may be one such family.

Reclaiming Trust

The word *tín* in Vietnamese and the Sanskrit word *shraddha* mean not only "trust" but also "faith" and "confidence." We use these three words—"trust," "faith," and "confidence"—almost interchangeably to describe the first strength. When we encounter abuse as children, we lose all three, both in ourselves and in others.

Trust or faith is the first of the Five Strengths and the first essential quality for a healthy life. As children, we absolutely need to develop trust that adults will care for us and provide us with a safe environment. Child victims of abuse lose faith in others, especially in adults. Adults are supposed to protect us, but instead, they become a frightening threat. These adults are most often our own family members—fathers, mothers, uncles, or elders in our communities.*

* Most of the perpetrators of child abuse (neglect, physical abuse, and sexual abuse) are family members. For example, in a 2011 child maltreatment report published by the US Department of Health and Human Services (HHS) and Child Protective Services (CPS), 80.8 percent of perpetrators were parents; perpetrators included siblings, other caretakers, and strangers: "Child Maltreatment 2011," ACF, accessed October 17, 2020, https://www.acf.hhs.gov/archive/cb/resource/child-maltreatment-2011).

According to research, in the United States one out of three women and one out of six men experience some form of sexual violence in their lifetime.* Transgender people are at an especially high risk of sexual violence. At the time of this book's writing, the good news is that the number of sexual assaults has declined over the past thirty years. However, more than 60,000 children are still reported to suffer from sexual abuse a year. Children as young as a few months old through the teen years are vulnerable. One out of four girls and one out of six boys will be sexually abused before they turn sixteen. Even as adults, one out of six women in the United States is a rape victim. Despite the widespread nature of these crimes in every country and culture, only a small percentage of them is reported to authorities.

Even when the abuse is from someone outside our immediate circle, we lose faith in our parents' ability to protect us. We expect our parents to protect us, but we see that they are unaware of what is happening to us. Ultimately, we may lose faith in ourselves, thinking, "I cannot protect myself. I am helpless." Having lost trust and confidence in ourselves and others, we may go headlong into a life of doubt, isolation, and fear.

Then there are the parents' responses to consider. Too many times, as in Claire's family, responses run along the lines of "Don't make up stories," "You must have enjoyed it," "Don't say anything to anyone; the social worker will take you away," and, perhaps most harmful of all, "Don't destroy this family." I have heard so many stories like this. Usually children don't say anything, but even when they do speak up, the adults often don't say anything helpful, and don't take immediate appropriate action, which deepens the mistrust, deepens the pain. The

---

* "Victims of Sexual Violence: Statistics," RAINN, accessed October 17, 2020, https://www.rainn.org/statistics/victims-sexual-violence.

caregivers' denial and inaction compound the child's mistrust, confusion, and pain. When abuse occurs in an institutional context, the responses of the authorities have the potential to help heal or add further harm. Therefore, it is crucial on the path of healing to acknowledge not only the original harm, but also the harm that occurs because it was not addressed in a timely and appropriate way.

Understandably, most survivors of sexual abuse have problems with trust in adult relationships. We may not trust our families, partners, institutions, or ourselves—we may even feel unsafe in our own bodies. Fortunately, our spiritual practice can help us to rebuild the foundation of trust first and foremost in ourselves. We don't have to wait for family or institutional change to begin healing; individual and collective healing can and must take place at the same time.

As we have seen in the first part of this book, mindfulness practice helps us come back to the body via the breath and helps us access our enormous power. Trauma victims may have certain breathing patterns and we may sense our body in atypical ways. We may hold tension in the body and suffer from post-traumatic stress. We may feel detached and dissociated (more on this in chapter 5, "Mindfulness as a Strength"). There are certain signs and symptoms of abuse that a skilled clinician can quickly decipher and help us understand. By developing mindfulness of the breath, the body, feelings, and thoughts, we can also aid our own healing process as we learn to be in our bodies and read our bodies' messages. This will take time and trust.

Modern psychotherapy provides several approaches that can help us understand ourselves, obtain some relief, and set up conditions for post-traumatic growth. Erik Erikson's stages of psychosocial development, which I learned in medical school, have remained with me as a useful framework that fits well with Buddhist practice. According to

Erikson, we develop in stages in life, from childhood through old age, moving through crises of opposing values, namely trust versus mistrust, autonomy versus shame and doubt, initiative versus guilt, industry or achievement versus inferiority, identity versus role confusion, intimacy versus isolation, generativity versus stagnation, and integrity versus despair. The first, most basic struggle is between trust and mistrust. The foundation of a person's lifelong health depends on the first stage of developing trust.

Unfortunately, if a child experiences abandonment, neglect, and/or abuse, the consequences can be devastating. Instead of developing trust, the child may develop mistrust, shame and doubt, guilt, fear, insecurity, confusion, and despair, which comprise an unhealthy emotional spectrum in all stages of psychosocial development. Depending on their personality and genetic makeup, some children may become frightened, needy, or overly anxious when they are left alone or in a new situation. Other children may shut down, becoming walled-off, hardened, resistant to relationships. Some conduct risky behaviors and disregard their own lives and safety. Some grow into adults who try not to attract sexual attention, while others develop high levels of sexual charisma, based on whatever behaviors in childhood helped them survive. Such extremes are signs of unhealthy development. Regardless of how the outer appearance of a person may manifest, deep in the core is a wounded child. Childhood trauma disrupts our development and prevents us from experiencing our own strengths fully.

A traumatic event may derail us and prevent us from completing a developmental stage, resulting in a reduced ability to move through further stages. When we understand the interbeing between these stages and the three times—past, present, and future—we can have confidence that these stages may be resolved successfully at a later time through spiritual practice. Western models of the mind tend to focus on individual experience, as if a person can exist in isolation, but Erikson's theory takes our community health into account and gives our social consciousness equal importance in a person's mental wellness and satisfaction in life. Indeed, a spiritual community may offer the second chance for individuals and families to heal and transform through our collective practice and collective awareness.

A Second Chance at Trust

How do we as individuals overcome such deep and widespread breaches of trust, so we can have full, loving, trusting relationships? To set up the right conditions for a safe and wholesome society, it is clear that we need to work collectively to prevent violence on the systemic and social level. Yet, we cannot wait for society to change in order to feel better in ourselves. We must address psychological and emotional scars that require attention. Throughout this book, we will explore how trauma survivors can build the experience of mental wellness into their lives with the Five Strengths. First, let us pay close attention to restoring the foundational strength of trust.

In the spirit of interbeing, we can recognize that these stages of psychosocial development do not take place in a linear fashion. They continue to take place throughout life, and any one stage can affect all other stages, positively or negatively.

In Buddhism, if trust has been damaged or broken at some point in our life, we can reestablish it with our spiritual practice. If our parents have failed to provide us safety and security, we can develop trust that we will be there to protect ourselves and to provide for our own needs. We can trust ourselves to not do what the perpetrator has done to us.

It's almost like we go through the stages of development all over again, but this time we take the initiative to equip ourselves with mindfulness, concentration, and insight. Now we are a teenager or an adult, and we can proactively make appropriate choices. Some therapists call this "reparenting."

Our spiritual life gives us this second chance. In fact, we have a new opportunity every time we are mindful of what is arising in us and around us. This is also a practice of being our own soul mate—remembering, knowing, and taking care of ourselves.

The Unspoken Trauma of Sexual Misconduct

Violations such as sexual harassment, assault, and rape are a deep pain in our world, which so many suffer from—yet we find it difficult to talk about these experiences. Usually, when there is a problem, we try to deal with it and find solutions, but sexual misconduct is an area that we can keep buried, unresolved and unaddressed. Recently, the #MeToo movement has helped to uncover the extent of sexual violence against women in our culture, and made it easier for all people to speak up about sexual violence. Young people are rapidly changing the culture, so that sexual abuse will be quickly reported and hopefully become less common. However, for several reasons, it is still very hard for children to tell even a trusted adult when someone is abusing them.

In the big picture, one reason childhood abuse of any type remains a social taboo is that its exposure threatens the trust that is the foundation of our society; it shatters our shared norms that create our reality. Childhood sexual abuse in particular destroys the social fabric of trust, which is why it is surrounded by stigma, shame, and silence.

The more powerful members of our human family are not supposed to take advantage of those who have less power or are more vulnerable. This is a treasured story in our society. We are not supposed to let our children get hurt. Men are supposed to respect women. Religious leaders are supposed to protect their congregations. Teachers are meant to have wholesome relationships with their students, and bosses at work should take care of their employees. Our governments are supposed to provide peace and prosperity. Yet our trust in those in power is all too often taken advantage of, undermined, and destroyed.

Another reason why children do not tell adults about abuse is that the children themselves may not know how to describe what is happening. As a child, I had actually seen my mother have sex with my old stepfather, but when my uncle molested me I did not put two and two together and see that his actions were sexual. I did not know what it was that he had been doing to me. Instinctively, it felt wrong. It felt frightening. I did not want to be in that situation again, but I could not articulate what was happening. I did not have the language to express it.

Children often keep abuse quiet because they feel that it is wrong, it is dirty, and it is their fault. Children also do not speak up because they are forbidden to do so, or threatened with harm if they do. Often abusers make their victims feel guilty and ashamed, as if they have brought it upon themselves: "You seduced me." "If you tell, you will be punished." "It is our secret!" Victims can come to believe, *Something about me causes these things to happen.* Or they may try to speak, and the adults in their lives may be too busy or preoccupied to show an interest, to listen; when there is a history of trauma in the family, as we have seen, parents may be in denial about what is happening, as the truth is too painful to contemplate.

Another reason children do not talk is that they may be frozen physically and mentally, so the memories are blocked out. In some cases, the children may deny the abuse even when approached by the adults. One young man told me that his granduncle sexually abused him and his sister when they were small. Eventually, his sister told their father, who sat down with him to ask him if it was true. The little boy replied, "No," and refused to talk further. To this day, he still does not know why he said that. The alienation and guilt that he has experienced with his sister and parents remain a source of implacable pain.

Abusers often have been victims themselves. Without appropriate care and healing, they may go on to abuse others, as the cycle of abuse is such that victims frequently become perpetrators, in a misguided attempt to resolve their trauma. Driven by shame and fear of humiliation, they may engage in cycles of denial, justification, rationalization, or minimization, which serve to cloud the truth of the damage they have suffered and have caused others.

In one family I know, two young girls who were cousins were exposed to pornography and molested repeatedly by a friend of the family who was living in their grandmother's house. One cousin tried to tell her mother, who retorted, "Shut up! Don't make up such horrible stories!" The little girl literally shut off and became sullen. When the other one grew into a teenager and finally told her own mother about the abuse, this parent lashed at her, "Why didn't you tell me earlier? You must have enjoyed it!" Reactions like this from adults are unfortunately common, and frequently the fear of meeting such a reaction is what holds young people back from seeking help.

We need to listen to children. I see again and again that adults find it challenging to listen to children because we do not even listen to ourselves. Many adults cannot bear the sound of a child crying. Instead of feeling compassionate, the sound arouses feelings of anger. Why is that? It could be that the sound triggers suppressed emotions, due to our own experience as children, being forced to cut off our feelings and stay quiet.

Unable to be in touch with ourselves, we do not know how to take care of ourselves, so when we become parents we cannot take care of our children. We need to say hello to the wounded children within us and invite them to speak. This will not only heal ourselves, but will also allow us to be present for the children in our lives.

🌸 *Practice: Listening to Your Inner Child*

Learning to listen deeply to yourself is a core practice of the Plum Village tradition. To take good care of yourself, you must not only listen to yourself in the present, but also go back and take care of the wounded child inside of you. Practice going back and listening to your wounded child every day. This child is here in the present moment, in every aspect of your life. You can heal them right now.

Be the big brother, big sister, mother, or father that you yearned to have. Embrace your own inner child tenderly.

First, establish yourself in your mindful breathing and in your body, as you did earlier in chapter 1. In all meditation practices, it is essential to listen to your breath and to your body at the beginning and throughout the session.

You can say, "My dear wounded child, I'm here for you, ready to listen to you. Please tell me all your suffering, all your pain. I am here, really listening."

Quiet repetition of these key words can help you hold your concentration until you can be in touch with your breath.

Breathing in, I listen to my in-breath.

Breathing out, I listen to my out-breath.

Listening to in-breath, out-breath

Breathing in, I am aware that my in-breath is ... [short, rapid, and loud or long, slow, and quiet]

Breathing out, I am aware that my out-breath is ...

Characteristics of in-breath, out-breath

Breathing in, I listen to my body.

Breathing out, I listen to my body.

Listening to body, smiling

Breathing in, I am aware that my body is ... [tired, tense, restless or relaxed, calm, at ease]

Breathing out, I am aware that my body is ...

Aware of the state of the body

Visualize yourself at the age when the trauma took place. As you follow your in-breaths and out-breaths, you can say,

My dear wounded child, I'm here for you. Please tell me about your suffering and pain. I am here, listening to you.

I'm here for you!

Remain anchored in your breath and your body, so that you may give your full attention and listen deeply to your inner child. Embrace that child mentally and physically and, as necessary, cry together with your inner child. Your mindful breathing and the relaxation of your body serve as the safe harbor for your child to name the injustice and to feel heard for the first time.

If you know how to go back to your inner child and listen like that every day for five or ten minutes, healing will take place immediately and will also unfold over time.

Undoubtedly, the practice of listening deeply to her inner child helped Claire to build trust in herself. Recently she told me at the end of a phone call, "Sister D, I want you to know that when things go bad, I don't tell myself that I should die anymore." It was the greatest gift she could offer me as her mentor.

Among us there are many people who have practiced like this, and after a period their suffering has diminished and transformed. We see the relationship between ourselves and others has become much better, much easier. We see more peace, more love in us.

Sexual Misconduct in Religious Organizations

A dear friend shared with me that her previous spiritual teacher asked her to sit on his lap. She was a grown woman, well-educated and strong-minded. Yet in that moment, she was overwhelmed by confusion and fear and obeyed him. She left this teacher and eventually found the Plum Village tradition, and through contact with a monastic tradition with integrity, she was able to regain her faith in spirituality. She experienced deep healing in her relationship with Thay and the monastic community.

Being sexually abused by people in your family or community is devastating, but to be sexually abused by a spiritual leader is undeniably more damaging. Wounded by your family of origin, you may come to spiritual life to find safety and healing. However, if you are hurt by your spiritual family, then you have nowhere else to go. You lose the rest of your trust and faith. If being abused by a family member made you lose faith in humanity, now you may lose faith in God or a higher power, or the purest, most sacred ideals of your life. Buddhist monks and nuns are definitely not Buddhas or gods, but people look up to us and turn to us in times of difficulty. As a result, it makes it even more devastating and destructive when we betray their confidence in us. Because we spiritual teachers represent the authority figure in the relationship, it makes some people even more hesitant to inform their parents or others if there is a breach of trust. Even if they do speak up, they may be met with denial.

Similar patterns may occur in any idealistic group with a charismatic leader, such as activist groups for the environment or human rights, or even a company where everyone holds the founder in high regard. People are attracted to the energy of fixing what's wrong, and they may bring their trauma from their family of origin to fighting for their cause, only to have their trauma further compounded when leaders betray their trust by acting without integrity. The more elevated the ideals, the harder the fall.

Due to several high-profile cases in the news, we now know that sexual misconduct in religious groups is more widespread than we ever suspected. Catholic priests abused altar boys for decades, but the victims could never talk about it—even when they grew up and it became clear that the church's focus was on preserving its power and protecting its priests rather than making reparations for the victims. If a case was brought to court, it would be settled quietly by the church and the offending priest might be sent away to a different parish, where he would continue to harm children. Child abuse in the Catholic Church has received the most extensive coverage, but groups in every tradition have had their faith broken.

It is vital to talk about sexual misconduct in spiritual communities to prevent it from occurring. As sexual abuse in spiritual organizations is such a common source of trauma, I would like to share briefly how my own Plum Village Community of Engaged Buddhism deals with sexual energy and prevents misconduct from occurring. Recognizing that sexual energy is inherent yet can be abused, we protect ourselves and others through the practice of "mindful manners" and precepts. Denying or suppressing our sexual energy only brings about tension and illness in our body and mind, and our training helps us acknowledge and recognize the presence of our sexual energy, taking care of it by protecting our six senses and guarding our thoughts, speech, and bodily actions with awareness.

Over the years, Thich Nhat Hanh frequently addressed the topic of sexual energy. Thay shared with his monastic students how he had learned to take care of his own sexual energy, channeling it to the breath and spiritual energy to benefit all people. As monastic practitioners, we strive to be honest and open, instead of denying our sexuality or fooling ourselves. Our monastic robes are modest and discreet, so as not to attract unwanted attention to ourselves. Our shaven heads also make us look more gender-neutral. All our daily activities help us cultivate our inner beauty and wholesome thoughts, focusing on cultivating a life of service and freedom.

We know that sexual activity or sexual attachment destroys the life of a monk or a nun, because we are no longer free to dedicate our life entirely to our spiritual practice and service. Therefore, we have many precepts addressing this topic from the most concrete to the most subtle, to raise awareness and prevent sexual energy from derailing us from reaching our aspirations.

Thich Nhat Hanh and the Plum Village community have revised the monastic codes for fully ordained monks and nuns, and these revised precepts are thoroughly pertinent to our modern time, including ways to deal with online abuse and sexual misconduct via phones, computers, electronics, and social media. In each Plum Village monastic community, we have Dharma discussions about our precepts monthly, and we recite our monastic precepts every two weeks. Our regular practice of precept recitation reinforces our mindful manners, so that when we cross a boundary, we are aware that we are crossing it. Instead of making excuses for it, we can reflect honestly: *Why am I doing this? Why am I making a minor transgression here?* This awareness can help prevent us from making a major transgression, which would terminate our monastic life.

As we train to become aware of our breathing, of our bodily sensations, of our thoughts and feelings, it becomes impossible to commit an act that's gross or harmful without being aware of it. Therefore, we have a chance to stop ourselves before a regrettable incident happens.

Sexual abuse is completely unacceptable in our monastic and lay community. In all our child and teenager programs, we never designate one monk to take care of the children; there are always monastic and lay brothers and sisters working together. If there is a scarcity of lay staff, then monastic sisters will take care of the children. Activities always take place in public spaces; we have a space designated for the children's program and another for the teens, with everyone in the program present. We are never alone with a child in a secluded place. When we give consultations to young people or adults, we make sure to sit in an open spot where others can see us. We encourage lay people to consider taking the basic precepts of the Five Mindfulness Trainings as a foundational moral code, which makes our society a safer place for everyone, especially children and families.

Over the years, I have gained deep appreciation for the monastic precepts, mindful manners, and regulations. Even when there is no danger of abuse occurring, our mindfulness practice sensitizes us to subtle interactions, and the precepts help me by serving as a mirror for me to see my mind. For example, there have been times when I have felt confined by the precepts, or have made small exceptions for myself; I have learned to use these rebellious thoughts and actions as bells of mindfulness, to alert me to the situation that I am in. Lo and behold, this usually happens when I experience an attraction to someone.

We may not be consciously aware of the attraction or subtly arising sexual energy, or we may deny it, but if we can see that certain mindful manners and precepts have been broken, then we will know that something is going on with us. Awareness of our own thoughts is essential. If we start to pay particular attention to somebody, think about somebody, approach somebody—these are red flags for us.

Unfortunately, when the passion or craving is stronger than our practice, it may overcome us. We have had some brothers and sisters disrobe because, as much as they might wish to pursue the monastic path, the sexual energy in them was overpowering. It is difficult to enter the monastic community, but leaving is always an option.

We have offered tea meditation as a ceremony of friendship for some of our brothers and sisters before they return to lay life. Once, when a sister had broken a precept and been asked to disrobe, Thay lovingly advised her, in front of all of us fully ordained nuns, "Even if you leave the monastic community to live a lay life, you still have to practice the Five Mindfulness Trainings." These are the five basic precepts any human can follow to have a happy life, which we will explore in part 3 of this book. "If you do not protect yourself and others," Thay continued, "you will suffer and cause your family and others to suffer." Living life as a layperson doesn't mean that we can do anything we want. We still need to practice.

Monastic brothers and sisters do sometimes fall in love with each other, and they may decide to leave the monastery together, but that is consensual on their part and not an abuse of power. When there is a romantic attachment between two individuals, the community tries to help them see their choices more clearly. If they transgress a major monastic precept and have sexual contact with each other, then they are requested to disrobe and leave the community immediately, but if communication is honest and trust is unbroken, they may leave with the community's best wishes for their shared future.

Trust in Mindfulness as a Process

When we have been through an experience that has left us traumatized, we can suffer from strong feelings of helplessness and powerlessness that do not seem to respond to logic. While we can understand the evolutionary basis for our fight-flight-freeze responses, there is still room for greater understanding of our neuroplasticity and our capacity for post-traumatic growth. Advances have been made in recent years in trauma research, leading to the development of therapies to treat PTSD, such as Somatic Experiencing and Eye Movement Desensitization and Reprocessing (EMDR) psychotherapy. Both these modalities work by helping practitioners transform their response to trauma. I encourage survivors who can access these therapies to try them. Unfortunately, access to high-quality therapy is an issue, and the number of trauma survivors relative to the resources available is overwhelmingly disproportionate.

In recent decades, mindfulness has been prescribed to address many issues, including anxiety and depression, both common effects of trauma. In the United Kingdom, for example, psychologists in the National Health Service have adopted mindfulness as a treatment for a number of symptoms of trauma. The wonderful thing about mindfulness as a path is that it can be practiced by anyone, anywhere. Mindfulness is self-awareness. Awareness is the foundation for change, transformation, and healing of one's own body, feelings, and thoughts. Self-awareness enables us to reconnect with our inner child's unmet needs, reestablishing trust and confidence that we can take care of our inner child from now on, thus empowering those of us who might have felt powerless to change for so long.

Practice: Acorn and Oak Tree Meditation

Let us visualize an acorn buried deep in the ground. With the right conditions of water, soil, and sunshine, it germinates and becomes a tiny oak sapling. With a lot more time, it becomes a magnificent, tall oak tree, giving wonderful shade to all those who sit beneath it.

Children are like young oak trees, beautiful and full of potential. You had all the right conditions to arrive where you are right now, and you continue to need all the right nourishment so that you may grow tall and strong and give shade to so many beings, including animals, plants, minerals, and humans.

Do you have a favorite kind of tree? Perhaps you have an actual favorite tree to practice with, which you can stand with as you practice this meditation. Take a moment to visualize yourself as an oak sapling or pine tree sprout or whatever kind of tree you like.

Breathing in and out, I see myself as a young plant, stretching in the sun, enjoying all the right conditions that are nurturing me: sunshine, rain, good soil, a lot of attention from nature, from the gardener.

Seeing myself as a young plant, enjoying favorable conditions

Breathing in and out, I enjoy being a young plant. May I be safe and happy. May I have all the right conditions so that I can take root deeper and deeper into the earth.

Enjoying being a young plant, taking deeper roots

For a tree to become tall and magnificent, it must have many roots, reaching down deep. Otherwise, the shallow roots cannot sustain it, and it will fall over or remain feeble. You were once young and dependent on your parents, teachers, and others to grow up, and like an acorn you possess the potential to become a mighty oak, strong in yourself and giving shade, sustenance, and protection to many. You can also learn to protect and care for yourself.

Following my in- and out-breaths, I see myself as an oak tree, stretching in the sun, enjoying all the conditions that nurture me: the sunshine, the rain, the good soil, and loving attention from myself as my own gardener now.

Seeing myself as an oak tree, enjoying favorable conditions

Following my in- and out-breaths, I enjoy being an oak tree. May I be safe and happy. May I take root deeper and deeper into the earth, and give shade to all around me.

Enjoying being an oak tree, taking deeper roots, and offering shade

If you feel inspired, you can reach out your arms to embrace your-self or your actual favorite tree.

As you go through your day, tune into your body and breath, know-ing you have everything you need for your healing. Trust in the process.

CHAPTER 4

Diligence as a Strength

In Buddhism, we speak of the five true powers, five kinds of energy ... faith, diligence, mindfulness, concentration, and insight. The five powers are the foundation of real happiness; they are based on concrete practices.

—THICH NHAT HANH, *THE ART OF POWER*

I had a groundbreaking experience while meditating in Plum Village, when I was a young novice. The community had purchased a farm in the early 1980s, which they had transformed into a rustic monastery. The buildings were made of big blocks of limestone from the region. I was sitting, meditating, with my monastic sisters, and in the middle of my meditation I opened my eyes and saw the stone wall before me. A thought arose, *How have I built this gigantic wall inside of me?* The wall seemed to be immovable, insurmountable.

I continued to follow my breathing as I sat there, staring at the wall. Tears streamed down my face continuously. Then, a few minutes later, another thought arose, that beneath the big blocks of stone, there were small stones wedged between them, and if even one small stone were to be removed, a little bit of light would pass through. *Then it would not be so dark anymore. There would be some light.*

I continued to sit, and another thought came to me: *Once one small stone is removed, it will be easier to remove a bigger stone.* Just sitting there with my mindful breathing and stable posture, slowly the realization came to me: *I can remove the blocks of stones slowly, and I do not have to remove all the stones. At a certain point, they will crumble by themselves because the foundation is no longer there to hold them up and keep them together. They will fall over by themselves, and then I can simply walk to the other side and enjoy the fresh air, the freedom.*

That was the first time I touched this wall of suffering inside of me and learned that the practice of meditation can help me to experience the lightness, peace, and freedom that were also within me. I did not have to transform all my suffering at once in order to be happy.

The Buddha's teachings of the Four Noble Truths and the Noble Eightfold Path can take a lifetime to learn and follow. People who believe in reincarnation might say that it takes many lifetimes! Yet the nature of the path is such that even if we only follow one aspect of it with sincerity and diligence, the rest of the path begins to open up in front of us. By meditating regularly every day, and giving ourselves dedicated time and space to heal, we will find ourselves receiving messages from our subconscious that will guide us toward transforming our suffering; we will develop deep insight or wisdom, the fifth of the Five Strengths. The wall of suffering within us is broken when just the first stone is removed; even if the structures that imprison us remain standing for a while, light can finally get through.

We begin the healing process with trust, but we need to apply ourselves to it with diligence. Diligence does not mean forcing. It means applying our energy in a wholesome way that is supportive of the health of our body and mind. We cannot force ourselves to heal any more than we can force a flower to bloom. We can only diligently provide the right conditions for it to grow and flourish.

How do we provide the best conditions for ourselves? The Buddha and many millions of practitioners since his time have developed and refined tools for leading a good life: the Four Noble Truths and the Noble Eightfold Path. Due to interbeing, in the Four Noble Truths we can find the Noble Eightfold Path and vice versa; we can start anywhere on the path and eventually all the directions will open up for us. For more about these timeless Buddhist principles, please read *The Heart of the Buddha's Teaching,* where they are beautifully taught in depth by Thich Nhat Hanh.*

The Four Noble Truths

Have you ever thought of suffering as being "noble"? The Buddha did, almost two thousand six hundred years ago. However, suffering is only noble if we know how to turn inward and find the way out. Otherwise suffering isn't noble at all. If we are hurt, we don't see any nobility in it. Mud alone is messy and sticky, but it can become beautiful lotus flowers if we know how to cultivate it skillfully.

Soon after he reached enlightenment, the Buddha spoke of the Four Noble Truths about suffering. Suffering can serve the noble purpose of leading to enlightenment when there is understanding into its nature. This is the art of suffering, the art of living. When I was a doctor, I told myself that I would never have to worry about being unemployed because there would always be sick people to treat wherever I went.

---

* See the Selected Resources on page 263.

Then when I became a nun, I realized that I would never have problems finding work in my monastic vocation either, because even though people may not be physically sick, they may be sad, or angry, or full of tension. There will always be a way to help people and develop my understanding of life.

A wonderful aspect of the monastic path that I have chosen is that I have a chance to take care of myself at a primary level, and it is from learning to understand and take care of my own body and mind that I may understand and help care for others more deeply and effectively. Through the application of mindfulness, I gain the necessary energy to heal and help others heal. The healer, the healed, and the healing are no longer separate entities. They inter-are. Before we can try to help others, it is important to be able to address our own suffering and trauma, to face it, smile with it, breathe with it, embracing it day after day until it is no longer an enemy that we have to run away from, or a pool of sorrow to drown in. Our suffering can be a friend and we can regard this friend with equanimity, tenderness, and love. Think of how animated and inspired you feel when you are in the presence of a true friend. Our suffering can give us the purpose, the energy, and the diligence to find a way to heal.

The First Noble Truth: Embracing Our Suffering

The First Noble Truth is awareness or mindfulness of the existence of suffering; it is the recognition and acknowledgment of the fact that we suffer. In fact, many of us suffer without realizing that we are suffering. For example, although we may be privileged enough to go shopping or to travel to other countries whenever we want, our consumption and diversions may actually be propelled by restlessness or discomfort.

Shopping or travel may serve to divert our suffering for a while, but they in turn water the seeds of more restlessness and discomfort in our consciousness that will manifest again, sooner or later, with stronger intensity.

When I was doing an internship in Kenya, I met Gladys, a young woman pregnant with a hydrocephalic child. She had had no prenatal care, and in her community, people did not go to see doctors unless it was a life-threatening situation. We had to do a Cesarean section because the child's head was enormous and could not be delivered otherwise. In hydrocephalus, the ventricle in the brain is blocked so the cerebrospinal fluid (CSF) cannot flow normally. As a result, the head becomes enlarged. The boy was born with a normal-sized body but with a triple-sized head. He looked grotesque. Gladys was only eighteen years old, and this was her first child.

When I first saw that child, I was startled for a second. Yet this young mother held her child ever so gently. She stroked her son's head that was so heavy, large, and deformed. Gladys knew that her child might not live very long, but she loved him while he was still there.

Can you hold your suffering in the same way, as your own child, as a part of yourself that you can care for, that you can be with?

Many people say, "I just want to forget my suffering," or "I just want to get rid of it." Yet, we cannot just let go of it that easily. Maybe we can forget it temporarily. Some pharmaceutical companies even try to invent drugs that can block certain memories or actually erase memories, like the protagonists in the film *Eternal Sunshine of the Spotless Mind*. However, it's not possible to erase certain memories selectively. When people medicate themselves to forget, they not only forget their painful memories but also the joyful ones. Do you really want to erase your memories?

Our spiritual practice is not for the purpose of forgetting, or of blocking our seeing or feeling. Instead, we have a spiritual practice in our daily life so that we can hold our pain and suffering, whether it is physical or mental, in the same way that the young woman Gladys could hold her child so tenderly and patiently. How she held that child!

The Second Noble Truth: The Causes of Suffering

The Second Noble Truth is about awareness or mindfulness of the causes of suffering, whether it is psychological, physical, and/or verbal; and the conditions that feed and perpetuate the suffering. The Buddha said that nothing can survive without food, and this is true of suffering. The practices of mindfulness, stopping, and deep looking, enable us to discover how we have been feeding our suffering. In this chapter we will also look at the practice of the Four Diligences, which empowers us to stop our suffering from perpetuating.

In contemplating the Four Noble Truths, we acknowledge the chief complaint that there is suffering, and then we reflect on the causes and conditions in order to confirm that there is a way out. In modern medicine, we call this "taking a history" of the patient. Just like in the First Noble Truth, taking a history of the patient starts out with their *chief complaint*, for example, "I've had a cough for three weeks now." Then the doctor proceeds to investigate the chronological progression of the patient's present illness from the first sign and symptom to the present. The doctor also asks about the patient's past medical history, family history, psychological history, and social circumstance, etc. Then the doctor may order some blood work and other lab tests to determine the causes in order to make the diagnosis. This is equivalent to the Second Noble Truth, identifying the causes and conditions of the dis-ease. The

Buddha pioneered this approach over two thousand five hundred years ago, and aptly, he was referred to as, "the King of Medicine."

As a young novice, when I first heard Thich Nhat Hanh giving his famous teaching "Pain is inevitable, but suffering is optional," it shook me to the core. A part of me felt indignant and rebellious, *What do you mean, suffering is optional? I have suffered all my life, and you say that it is optional?* I felt that Thay's statement undermined and trivialized the trauma that I had endured in my life.

Nevertheless, something deep inside me knew that my teacher was right. Learning to be more aware of the workings of my mind, I saw more clearly how my way of thinking, speaking, and behaving fed my own suffering and perpetuated it. Even if physical or emotional pain only takes place in a single moment in time, the suffering that results from our negative interpretations and unmindful reactions toward that pain is continuous, relentless, unbearable, and long-lasting. I began to have insight into my state of PTSD.

I had identified myself by my suffering for many years, so it was not easy to "just let it go." To be able to embrace suffering is a process of getting to know its roots, of living in harmony and in non-fear with the past, the present, and the future. Suffering is an art that can be learned and mastered. The art of suffering can bring about deep appreciation for life as well as profound peace, joy, and love for ourselves and other beings. Thus, the art of suffering and the art of happiness are not two separate entities. They inter-are.

The Buddha explained that we suffer because of our wrong views and wrong thinking. The phenomena that we experience in our lives are impermanent and without a discrete "self," but because we think of them as permanent and with a self, we suffer. When something feels good, we want to be with it all the time, and we suffer when we must be apart from it. When something feels bad, we want to reject it, and we suffer when we must face it. Therefore, suffering is not intrinsic in the phenomena themselves. Suffering results from our attachment or aversion to experiences.

The Third Noble Truth: Happiness Is Entirely Possible

The Third Noble Truth is about the cessation of suffering, in other words, the presence of true happiness. Many of us live as if in the here and now, only plans, projects, worries, regrets, and fears are possible, but not happiness. We believe superstitiously that happiness belongs to a distant past or to a dreamy future, but not to the present moment.

The Third Noble Truth is equivalent to making a *prognosis* in modern medicine, which is the predicted outcome of the illness, depending on the patient's general health condition and the *diagnosis*, whether it is lung cancer, COVID-19, or a simple cold. Then the doctor proposes a *treatment plan* for the patient. In the Third Noble Truth, the Buddha was fully confident and optimistic in declaring, "Cessation of ill-being is entirely possible. Ill-being can be transformed one hundred percent." Thus, suffering can be transformed into happiness. This prognosis affirms that indeed, happiness belongs to the present moment, right here and right now, if you comply to the treatment.

The treatment that the Buddha prescribes is the Noble Eightfold Path, which leads to complete transformation and healing. In the sutra known as The Buddha's Diagnosis, the Buddha further asserted that the Noble Eightfold Path has the capacity to prevent the illness from ever recurring. In the past, many Buddhist scholars misinterpreted the Four Noble Truths as pessimistic, that the Buddha claimed this world is full only of suffering; everything is suffering and there is no way out of it. However, as we look deeply into all Four Noble Truths, we see that they are remarkably scientific and optimistic.

The Fourth Noble Truth: The Way Out of Suffering into Happiness via the Eightfold Path

The Fourth Noble Truth is about the concrete practices of the Noble Eightfold Path: right mindfulness, right concentration, right view, right thinking, right speech, right bodily actions, right livelihood, and right diligence. If we practice the "right" approach in these eight areas, we are bound to come out of suffering.

The Four Noble Truths together with the Eightfold Path can be approached as a kind of Buddhist Twelve-Step program, although they offer an even deeper transformation of those habits of mind that spark suffering in us. They provide concrete practices to transform the addiction to and perpetuation of suffering at its root, guaranteeing the fruit of happiness in every moment we are practicing them. As Thich Nhat Hanh has pointed out, whether we follow the teachings of the Four Noble Truths and the Noble Eightfold Path is a choice-point leading to suffering or happiness, or as "nutriments" feeding suffering or happiness. In this light, the Four Noble Truths are astonishingly sober, asserting that we have agency in our happiness or suffering, which we can cultivate with a sense of purpose and intention.

Mindfulness is the energy that enables us to wake up and listen to the cry of our own suffering, embracing it tenderly the way of a mother holding her child in her arms, to acknowledge our own discomfort and to find its causes, so we can remedy the problem and bring about relief and well-being. If we know how to deal properly with suffering, we will suffer less and we will be able to transform it into understanding, love, healing, and happiness. We can acknowledge the value and usefulness of suffering, and we do not have to run away from it anymore.

It is important to practice the steps of the Noble Eightfold Path in our daily lives. We can experience great insights, but if we don't have a way to practice in our daily life, these insights may not become realized. Then there is a danger that we may see ourselves as hypocritical or helpless and lose the confidence to keep walking on the path.

There's the saying "Ignorance is bliss." It is more painful when we see the situation we are in and we cannot change it. For example, most of my life, before I woke up to the depth of my trauma, I suffered, but I was largely unconscious of its source. Then I went to my first mindfulness retreat. I came back more aware, but unable to maintain the practice I had learned on retreat since I had returned to the daily stress of a young doctor's job. Actually, my pain felt more excruciating, because I had become keenly aware of my situation. At that point, we cannot be in basic survival mode any longer, and we know that we are not being true to ourselves. It is painful to clearly see our dilemma in this light for the first time. The Four Noble Truths and the Noble Eightfold Path offer us a way out.

The Four Diligences: Handling Seeds Emerging from Store Consciousness

Together with the Noble Eightfold Path, in Buddhism we have an abundance of teachings that help us heal our suffering. For trauma survivors, the Buddhist psychology idea of seeds of consciousness can be very powerful and liberating. Our consciousness is like a storehouse of possibilities, which are like seeds in storage, so we call it "store consciousness." This corresponds with our subconscious mind in Western psychology. Embedded within our store consciousness are various kinds of wholesome and unwholesome seeds. The wholesome seeds lead to thoughts, speech, and bodily actions that nurture life, peace, harmony, happiness, and inclusiveness. On the other side of the spectrum, unwholesome seeds lead to destruction, discrimination, conflict, and division.

When a seed held in store consciousness manifests at the more easily perceived level of the conscious mind, or what we often call "mind consciousness," it is referred to as a mental formation, such as joy, love, desire, depression, etc. For example, if you tend to be depressed, meditation may help you identify this tendency as a seed of depression in your store consciousness. It may be a seed you have inherited from your ancestors.

The practice of the Four Diligences aims at the mental formations emerging from store consciousness into mind consciousness as soon as they start to manifest. This is a process of mindful consumption, an intake of not just concrete things like food, but of all kinds of sense impressions and sensations. In our daily life, we continually bring images, sounds, conversations, tastes, touch, thoughts, perceptions, etc. into our store consciousness; even a smell can trigger a certain memory. A cologne or perfume can bring back the image of someone you have not seen for years. A food smell can make you think of Grandma's cooking. And a thought itself can trigger an entire physiological stress response, as in the case of post-traumatic stress disorder (PTSD).

Preventing the negative seeds from taking root in our consciousness requires us to stop and remain calm. It's similar to not aggravating an already angry dog who's ready to bite us. Some years ago, while living at Magnolia Grove Monastery in Tennessee, I would often go out jogging alone. One day, three dogs started barking aggressively from their front yard as soon as they saw me. I stood still, and they crossed the road, still barking and circling me. The biggest of the three dogs jumped up on me, up to my waistline, smearing saliva all over my brown pants. The medium-size dog circled and barked continuously, but it did not jump on me. The smallest dog just stood by and barked at me from a short distance. The whole time, I just stood still and breathed. Occasionally, I would say softly to the dogs, "It's okay. It's okay, my dear."

After a while, the smallest dog became quiet. Then he started to bark at the other two. It was clear that he was communicating with the others. Then he took a few steps away from me. The other two dogs also began to back off. Then all three ran back to their front yard. They continued to bark at me a while longer, but mildly. I remained standing still until they had returned to their house, and then I slowly continued on my way.

As long as I remain calm and nonreactive, I have learned that aggressive dogs will eventually walk away. I have also learned to be calm in frightening situations with people, and it has saved my life several times. If we react with fear and hatred, our reaction may further sow the seeds of aggression and ruthlessness in humans as well as in dogs, while our energy of stillness and calm makes them return to their original quiet state. This energy of peacefulness is not passive, but extremely active. It is a nonviolent approach to a violent situation, and it may not come naturally to us; we need to understand how it works and train for it. The Four Diligences help us generate this energy.

The First Diligence: Maintain and Support Positive Mental Formations

The First Diligence is to keep a positive state of mind. If the mental formations are wholesome, then we want to keep them in the mind consciousness for as long as possible, which in turn nurtures these particular wholesome seeds in the store consciousness. Actively recognizing the conditions that help these wholesome mental formations to manifest, we can maintain these conditions and create further advantageous conditions for them. For example, if we know that a certain group of friends usually makes us feel engaged and positive, then we would want to create opportunities to interact with them more frequently.

The Second Diligence: Help More Positive Seeds to Manifest

The Second Diligence is that if the wholesome seeds have not yet manifested, then we help create conditions for them to manifest. When wholesome mental formations manifest in the landscape of our mind consciousness, the quality of our lives improves. We can contribute positively to our families and society. This is also a practice of planting flowers in the garden. The more trees and flowers we plant, the less space there is for weeds to grow. We actively cultivate the wholesome seeds and give them room to grow.

The Third Diligence: Return Negative Mental Formations to Store Consciousness

The Third and Fourth diligences are directed at the unwholesome seeds that are in our store consciousness. If negative seeds manifest in the mind consciousness as negative and unwholesome mental formations (such as jealousy, greed, anger, and competitiveness), then we do what we can to bring them back to our store consciousness.

We can do this by inviting the energy of mindfulness to arise, to embrace the negative emotions and calm them down. This is done through mindful breathing, walking meditation, abdominal breathing, sitting meditation, and so forth. For example, we can practice with "Breathing in, I am aware of anger arising in me. Breathing out, I smile and relax my anger." Or, "Breathing in, I am aware that I have a strong perception about somebody. Breathing out, am I sure that it is correct?"

Of course, there are situations when we need to act quickly and decisively. When a house is burning down, it is essential to extinguish the fire and to save whatever we can. Only afterward would we try to find the cause of the fire. Similarly, when there is a storm of emotion, we should try to protect our body and mind from being burned up or destroyed by it. Mindful breathing and the simple recognition of our strong emotions enable us to master our emotions more promptly and effectively. Once we have a calm body and clarity of mind, then we can look deeply into the triggering factors of our strong emotion. Each time we are able to calm down, return an unwholesome mental formation back to the store consciousness, and understand its root, the seed will become weaker. Eventually it will manifest with less frequency and intensity.

Another practice is "changing the song," giving rise to a positive thought, to a feeling of empathy and understanding, to right view and right thinking. We can direct our attention to something positive that is also available in the present moment.

The Fourth Diligence: Keep the Negative Seeds from Arising

The Fourth Diligence is directed at the unwholesome seeds in our store consciousness that have not yet manifested in mind consciousness. They can then remain dormant. Recently, a teenager told me, "I just don't like to play violent video games anymore. It doesn't make me feel good anyway." She stopped subjecting herself to stimuli that she found harmful, and thus she was able to prevent the negative cascade of reactions from arising within them in the first place. With awareness of how our body feels in certain situations, we will be able to stop feeding the negative seeds that still lie dormant in our consciousness.

Why is it so essential to keep the negative seeds from arising or from feeding them? Through the power of affinity, manifestation of some unwholesome seeds may trigger a host of other unwholesome seeds, which impede the growth, restoration, and healing of our body and mind. Then, when a highly stressful situation takes place, like a pandemic, a severe illness, or the death of a loved one, these unbeneficial seeds may flood our mind consciousness, impairing our judgments, affecting severely our speech and behaviors, and aggravating preexisting conditions. For example, since the advent of COVID-19, many more people have reported suffering from PTSD, depression, and anxiety. The incidences of domestic violence, sexual abuse, overdoses, suicide, and homicide have increased.* All these phenomena reflect how unequipped we are as individuals and as a society in taking care of our trauma. Knowing that such pain will continue to affect us long after the pandemic has passed, we can be determined to apply the Four Diligences in our daily life so that we may have a greater capacity for transformation and healing.

---

* Mark É. Czeisler, et al. "Mental Health, Substance Use, and Suicidal Ideation During the COVID-19 Pandemic—United States, June 24–30, 2020." Centers for Disease Control and Prevention. August 13, 2020. Accessed October 29, 2020. https://www.cdc.gov/mmwr/volumes/69/wr/mm6932a1.htm.

🌸 Practice: Changing the Song

This practice relates to the Four Diligences, watering the positive seeds and not the negative seeds that have arisen or not yet arisen. When a song starts playing that we don't like, we can change the song. If we notice that negative mental states are being watered or triggered, we can consciously change the scene. For example, if you are watching a movie that has violence or sexual abuse, and it's making you cry or feel sick, you do not have to sit there and endure it. Just because such scenes have been normalized as entertainment does not mean they are indeed normal. Change the channel. Turn the television or the computer off. Leave the room or the theater. Go for a walk or sit quietly to calm your emotions. And remember, you have every right to avoid that sort of triggering experience in the future.

CHAPTER 5

Mindfulness as a Strength

How can anyone ever tell you that you are anything less than beautiful?

How can anyone ever tell you that you are anything less than whole?

How can anyone ever fail to notice that your life is a miracle, that you are deeply connected to all lives?

—PLUM VILLAGE SONG

As abused children, we may look at our body in a negative way and say to ourselves, "I have done something wrong. My body is dirty. My body is shameful." Consequently, as adults we may carry our body without acceptance, love, or confidence. I have heard many people say, "I hate my body," or "I feel alienated in my own body."

At one of our large retreats, a young woman named Jane shared that when she took her seat for sitting meditation and closed her eyes, she saw her body as gigantic, with her hands especially out of proportion. She asked me if it was normal to feel like that. Through her responses to my questions, even though she did not talk about it directly, I recognized that she had been abused as a child, and she had adapted an "out-of-body experience" as a coping mechanism. When something occurs that is so painful it is unacceptable, the mind distances itself from the body and leaves it behind, so that it does not have to experience the body's pain and humiliation. We may not have such a dramatic experience as Jane's, but dissociative experiences of this nature are common among trauma survivors.

People going through this kind of experience describe it as their mind or spirit floating out of the body. From above, the mind can look down at the body going through torture or abuse, but the mind itself is distant and numb to suffering. It is a coping mechanism that allows the mind to not feel the excessive pain in the body during the traumatic incident. Unfortunately, many of us continue to stay outside of our body even after the abuse is long past. We are not in touch with our body; we see our body from a distance. Therefore, we cannot love, take care of, and be affectionate and kind to our own body.

Some of us have deep pain that we carry but paradoxically cannot feel. We may cut our wrists and arms and legs to restore a sense of feeling and relief—at the same time, causing further harm to the body. So wrapped up in our painful feelings and so out of touch with our own body, we cut ourselves in order to feel our body, to feel that we are connected to it and have some measure of control over it. Other self-harming behaviors include scratching, hair pulling (which I did when I was a teen), eating disorders, and excessive exercise. We may also turn to drugs and alcohol to feel better in our bodies, even when we know they are not a solution.

I advised Jane to learn and practice breathing mindfully, to help her join her mind to her body in a healthy, wholesome way. Just as in the breathing practice in chapter 1, we began by getting in touch with our in-breaths and out-breaths, by closing and opening our hands in time with our breathing. Our breathing, as we know, is a sensitive indicator of the movement of our mind. The breathing pattern changes when we have different kinds of feelings and emotions, so to be in touch with and harmonize the breath is to help harmonize the body as well as the mind, so that the mind can dwell within the body. We can train to get our awareness back into our bodies.

I encouraged Jane to stay within her body through her mindful breathing, and to stay grounded in reality. If she could not mentally scan her body with her eyes closed, if she felt that her hands were gigantic again, then she could open her eyes to look at her hands and hold one hand in another, to verify that they were indeed very much in proportion with the rest of her body. This would help train her mind to come back and dwell within the reality of the body instead of leaving it and perceiving it with distortion. Mindful breathing became a bridge for her to reconnect her mind with her body, and thus reconnect her with herself.

Mindfulness Is Meditation in Action

Why does mindfulness have such a profound effect on the mind and body? Meditation existed long before the advent of Buddhism, as much a part of many other religious traditions as contemplation and prayer. However, mindfulness meditation as a practice is unique to Buddhism. In the Pali canon, the Buddha frequently exhorted his monastic and lay disciples to practice mindfulness, as seen in the Discourse on the Full Awareness of Breathing and the Four Establishments of Mindfulness.* In his research of the Pali canon, Thich Nhat Hanh found that the word for "mindfulness" (*sati* in Pali, *smirti* in Sanskrit) was used two hundred times more frequently than the word for "meditation" (*dhyana*). While the four stages of dhyana are discussed and emphasized in some

---

* The texts of these are in Thich Nhat Hanh, *Breathe! You Are Alive: Sutra on the Full Awareness of Breathing* (Berkeley, CA: Parallax Press, 1996).

later meditation traditions, the Buddha's basic teachings on meditation focus on stopping and deep looking. These two elements of meditation, like two wings of a bird, are specific and unique to Buddhism, and they are embedded in mindfulness.

You may think that meditation requires a specific time and place, such as sitting down on a cushion. In fact, mindfulness as a meditation can take place anywhere, anytime, and all the time. In particular, for the person who is recovering from trauma, simply sitting still for meditation can be a challenge; the moment we sit and close our eyes, memories, images, and intrusive thoughts may prevent us from following our in-breaths and out-breaths, our body may feel far from relaxed, and our mind may be neither clear nor calm. Jane's story is just one example of how traditional seated meditation can be a challenge.

Applying mindfulness in daily life helps trauma survivors because it helps us get in touch with ourselves at a physiological and neurological level, with an attitude of self-compassion toward our stress and suffering. I invite you to consider that wherever you are and whatever you are doing, it can be a meditation, whenever you come back to the awareness of your breathing and of your body. Mindfulness is meditation in action, meditation in the present moment.

The Functional Freeze Response

Our physiological response to a stressful situation is known as the "fight, flight, freeze, or faint response." Most of us are aware of the physical manifestations of "fight or flight" and we may even be aware when we are experiencing them in our daily lives. Our heart rate, blood pressure, and respiratory rate increase. We argue, we avoid. We fight, we run away. The freeze response is less well known, but it is the oldest survival mechanism of all. When fighting our way out or running away from a threatening situation seems impossible, our autonomic nervous system activates the freeze response as the last resort. Fear-induced fainting is an extreme stress survival response to an inescapable threat.

For example, when a mouse is being played with by a cat, it knows it cannot fight, so it tries to save itself by running for its life. If it cannot do that, the freeze response will automatically take over, causing the mouse to faint or literally drop dead. In that way, if the cat were to eat the mouse, the unconscious mouse would not have to feel the pain of being eaten alive. Another advantage of this freeze mechanism is that it increases the mouse's chance of survival: when the cat sees the mouse has stopped running and is lying unconscious, it may no longer be interested in playing with the mouse or eating a thing that is already dead. The cat might walk away, and then the mouse would wake up at a certain point. In this case, it may run for its life, or literally shake off the experience, recover completely, and move on.

As human beings, we may faint during a traumatic episode, or our mind may distance itself from the body in an out-of-body experience, and the body may be frozen in fear and unable to move. What psychologists call the "functional freeze response" can help us survive, to shield us from further pain and suffering. Afterward, however, we may not have the chance to calm down and process the experience properly.

With sexual trauma, moreover, as we discussed previously, usually there is a deep vein of social shame that keeps us from being able to speak about our pain and get help. We may not be able to access the social support that is essential for managing our stress responses. We may not have the emotional space to take care of our wounds properly. We may need to pretend to be fine, or we may cover up the experience, as if it were all normal. We may check out, shut down, or dissociate from our body to avoid feeling our pain. We may deny it happened, or hide it from our own family members, friends, and even ourselves. After all, whether we are children or adults, there are roles, duties, and responsibilities to perform as soon as we can get back on our feet.

The terms "functional freeze" and "out-of-body experience" both describe phenomena in which the mind is separated from the body. All of us experience this occasionally, when our body is here but our mind is wandering or fantasizing elsewhere. It becomes maladaptive and destructive when our mind resorts to it frequently, habitually, or as an ongoing state.

In an abusive situation when traumas may happen repeatedly, we may get stuck in a state of chronic stress. We cannot fight back or run away, so we freeze. This coping mechanism becomes maladaptive when we continue to stay in this frozen state mentally, long after the event that caused the initial stress is over. Having been abused as children, we may grow up, have relationships and families, carry out responsibilities, pursue goals and ambitions, but something inside us has frozen. We move through life mechanically. Unlike the fainted mouse that gets up and moves on, we remain deadened and frozen inside, alienated from our own body and life energy, out of touch with our feelings, disconnected with what is important in our life. We may be in this state of "functional freeze" without being aware of it, and those who are close to us may sense something is wrong, but not be able to pinpoint what it is.

Common Coping Mechanisms and Controlling Behaviors

The same unsafe situation may trigger a fight or flight reaction in some of us, while it may trigger a total shutdown in others. Therefore, understanding the trauma response is critical to our healing. We also need to keep an open mind about the different manifestations of trauma and the coping mechanisms that we may employ, consciously or unconsciously. Depending on our genetic makeup, personality, and background, we may use drugs or alcohol, or the more socially acceptable addictions to food, sex, or work, etc., to soothe, suppress, or escape our feelings. These are all methods we adopt to cope with pain. Therefore, it is essential to identify how we control ourselves in different areas of our lives and see if a behavior is truly beneficial or if it may be harmful.

We can talk about just a few of the common mechanisms here, but I invite you to apply what I say to any behavior you identify as harmful. Some of the most common coping mechanisms I encounter are around food. Some may control their stress through either overeating or under-eating. Unhealthy eating patterns tend to reflect a negative coping mechanism for trauma. We may use food as a means to control our life, because otherwise we feel out of control over our life. It feels like a way of dealing with insurmountable suffering. Eventually, this controlled eating may develop into an eating disorder.

There are two extremes. One is to eat in order to *soothe* strong feelings; this is eating according to what we feel, as in the case of binge-eating and bulimia. The other is to starve ourselves to *repress* strong feelings; this is controlling what we feel, as in anorexia nervosa. Both mechanisms often relate to a negative body image, which further creates a vicious cycle. Controlled eating is similar to cutting, picking the skin, or pulling hair, in that we feel helpless in our situation, so at least we can do something to our own body to feel in control.

Eating meditation can help us reestablish a healthy relationship with food, the way we learn to reestablish a healthy relationship with our body by nurturing and loving the body. Similarly, we can heal our relationship with food, receiving food with gratitude in order to nourish our body, instead of eating it but hating it, hating ourselves, hating our sense of hopelessness and being powerless.

In the area of intimacy, we may find that we use sex to control our feelings. We may avoid sex completely or get recklessly involved in sex. It may give us a sense of being in control, but in fact reflects how out of control our pain and confusion are, perpetuating our suffering further. For example, the mind may fool itself into thinking, "I have control over my body. I choose to have sex or not, whereas before I did not have a choice."

Some may manifest maladaptive behaviors through work. We become workaholics in order to escape from our feelings and from the painful relationships that we may have in the present. Others may become depressed and incapacitated, staying home and feeling shame, guilt, and worthlessness year after year.

❧ Practice: Eating Meditation

Eating is an activity that most people do at least three times a day, and it can become a rich opportunity for meditation with stopping and deep looking. While cooking or preparing your food, you can stand upright and relaxed, smiling and returning to your natural in-breaths and out-breaths. All your senses are nourished by food and the act of eating. The sight and the smell of the food can nourish you already.

Take just enough food or perhaps a little less than you need; you can always refill your plate if you are still hungry. Notice the gap between what you need and what you want. Give rise to the empathetic thought that many people in the world go to sleep hungry each night. How fortunate you are that your empty plate will soon be filled!

Allow yourself to have at least twenty minutes to eat. As you eat, to savor the taste and texture of your food fully, try eating in silence for at least the first five or ten minutes. Eating quickly and talking while eating can cause indigestion and overeating. Glucose from the digested food needs about twenty minutes to get into the bloodstream and to reach the brain in order to signal that you are full. When you eat fast, glucose does not reach the brain fast enough, and so you keep eating. By the time you feel full, you have actually overfed yourself.

Eating slowly helps you to enjoy the food and also helps you to eat less. Monks and nuns hardly ever need to be on a diet, because we eat slowly, we enjoy the food, and we know when we are just full. There are millions of diet fads to maintain a healthy weight, but I have discovered that mindful eating is the best way to keep our weight under control, while enjoying our food deeply and, at the same time, healing our relationship with food.

Following your breathing as you chew the food can help you to stay calm and relaxed. Putting down your fork or spoon on the table while you are chewing also helps your mind to focus on the food that is in your mouth instead of automatically preparing for the next bite already. By chewing properly and without hurrying, you are giving your stomach and small intestines less work to do.

Multitasking while eating by watching television or working on your computer, you do not consume only the food but also the images that are shown on television and messages on the computer screen. You consume images and sounds. You consume thoughts and plans. You consume worries, anger, disappointment, and others' feelings, instead of being present to your own body's healing. It's no mystery why you may feel sick after you eat, or you do not feel nourished at all, because you have consumed more toxins from thoughts and feelings than nutriments from the food itself.

In our practice centers, we serve our food in silence, walk quietly to the dining area, sit down together, and wait for three sounds of the bell and the reading of five contemplations on eating before we begin eating. Eating slowly and mindfully in this way, paying attention to how we consume repairs the damage we have caused to our body with years of rushing and stress.

Dissociation and the Role of the Breath in Reconnecting

I met a woman a few years ago who'd had breast cancer and undergone a bilateral mastectomy—both of her breasts had been removed. We met at a Day of Mindfulness I had helped to facilitate at her workplace. At the end of the day, she said to me, "You know something, Sister D? Since I had my surgery, for seven years now, I have not looked at my body from the neck down." When she looked in the mirror, she only looked at her face. She could not look at the rest of her body.

Her story is not unusual. Many of us who have had something unwanted happen to our body cannot bear to see the effects. We may notice that we develop habits of avoiding the evidence of anything we don't want to think about. How many of us say we don't like the look of ourselves in photographs, once we grow older or our bodies have changed? Social shame may combine with our inner trauma and prevent us from fully loving and healing ourselves.

It is important to realize that these dissociative responses to stress or trauma are automatic, triggered by the sympathetic nervous system in the case of the fight or flight response and the parasympathetic nervous system with the freeze response. As victims, we may blame ourselves for not being able to fight back effectively. Running away or being frozen on the scene may trigger shame in us later on. We must understand that our nervous system had made that decision automatically in order for the optimal outcome, which is our survival and subsequent safety.

A way to heal this shame or blame is to acknowledge our nervous system's wisdom and to thank our body for having made that choice in response. The proof of success is that we are still here. Then, we can take the next step of healing ourselves by acknowledging that we are now safe and secure. Slowly, we train ourselves not to resort to fight, flight, or freeze when new situations arise. We learn to respond proactively instead of reacting automatically out of habit.

In chapter 2, we learned the practice of listening to our other brains, including the body brain, the heart brain, the lung brain, and the gut brain. This is a proactive way of resetting our autonomic nervous system, which is often on alarm mode in survivors of trauma. In order to trigger the fight or flight response, the sympathetic nervous system activates the heart, the lungs, and the skeletal muscles. With the awareness of the messages from our heart and lungs, we can help calm down this activation with mindful breathing and relaxing the body, thoughts, and feelings. We can stop receiving further inputs that trigger this response.

The parasympathetic nervous system, on the other hand, is responsible for shutting down, collapse, dissociation, or passing out. It is characterized by massive down-regulation of the autonomic activation. While these are involuntary responses, we can help shift them at a base level by committing ourselves to self-care: being more physically active in life, nourishing ourselves with right view and positive thinking, establishing a healthy diet, and reaching out for meaningful connection with family members and friends.

🌸 Practice: Befriending Ourselves with the Breath

When we learn to simply come back to the breath, moment to moment, we are training our mind to come back to be with the breath, to see whether it's shallow or rapid, of if the touch of the breath can only be felt at the nostril level or the throat level. We observe without judgment, kindly, and gradually we learn to identify when our breathing is stressed. When we breathe in a very shallow way, we know we're under stress. We learn to be with that, placing our hands on our chest, on our belly, as we practiced in chapter 2, and we just breathe. Be with the breath, be with the body, and come back to the life that's flowing in the breath and the body.

To be with the breath and the body can be very threatening, scary, alienating for many of us, because we have deserted ourselves for so long. Slowly and patiently, we befriend our body, to recognize that the body is the mind, the mind is the body—they inter-are.

What about our sadness, where do we find it? It's in the heaviness of our chest, in the fatigue of our body. Where do we find anger? In the trembling of our hands, in our quickened heartbeat. Every emotion manifests in our body. Our body is a manifestation of our mind. So to take care of our body and our breathing is to take care of our mind and our emotions, such as sadness, despair, or confusion. Instead of habitually feeling alienated and frightened by the body, we gradually feel that it is comforting and empowering to be in the body through the practice of mindful breathing, scanning the body, relaxing the body, and sending it love.

You may like to practice breathing here again like we did in chapter 2, befriending your breathing and sending yourself extra love.

Breathing in, I befriend my in-breath

Breathing out, I befriend my out-breath.

Befriending in-breath and out-breath. Hello!

Breathing in, I observe my in-breath

Breathing out, I observe my out-breath.

Observing in-breath and out-breath. I see you!

Breathing in, I follow my in-breath from beginning to end.

Breathing out, I follow my out-breath from beginning to end.

Following in-breath and out-breath. I'm with you!

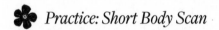 *Practice: Short Body Scan*

As you get more in touch with the physical body, you develop the ability to mentally scan your body from the top of your head to the soles of your feet. Lying down in a comfortable position on the floor or other flat surface, allow yourself to relax, close your eyes, and move your awareness of your bodily sensations through your body from part to part. There is nowhere to go, nothing to do but be present with your body and give it your attention.

There are guided body scans on the Plum Village app and other mindfulness apps that you might like to try. As we scan through each part of our body, we can breathe into it, acknowledge it, and send gratitude and affection to it. If any part of the body is in pain or numbness, we can breathe into that part for a while longer, as if we were massaging it with our mindful breathing. We are sending our awareness to the painful or frozen parts of our body and mind. This practice is to acknowledge that pain or numbness is there, and to send the message to our body that we are now present for our body and that we care to understand our situation better and to take care of it as our beloved.

Before you practice, you may like to say the *gatha* below.

This body is the body of my ancestors,
    containing all wisdom and potential for liberation.
May I live with full awareness of my body,
    so that healing and transformation may take place every
    moment.

❁ *Practice: Guided Deep Relaxation*

Deep relaxation is an opportunity to come back to be in contact with our body. We recognize the wonders of our eyes, our hands, our lungs, and everything else. We also become more aware of the tension and pain in the body, which perhaps originate from the body but may also come from difficult circumstances and sadness over the years. Our body is a manifestation of our mind, and if there is sadness and pain in the mind then it will manifest and remain in the body. The mind may be invisible and abstract, but with regard to the body, we can see, hear, smell, taste, touch, and perceive it. Therefore, we learn to befriend and relax each part of our body, knowing that when the body can be relaxed and at ease, the mind naturally becomes lighter and more peaceful, providing optimal conditions for our healing.

Moreover, when we focus on strong emotions such as anger, anxiety, or depression, it can feel vague, overwhelming, and even paralyzing. Yet if we can recognize how these strong emotions manifest in the body, they become more concrete and perceivable, and we can relax and send love to the parts of the body that are tense or painful. As a result, awareness of the body and the practice of deep relaxation can heal body and mind simultaneously. We can practice body awareness and relaxation throughout the day, anywhere and anytime. Even if we practice deep relaxation for five to ten minutes before we go to sleep, when we wake up, and then after lunch, the benefits will already be evident.

You can use this guided deep relaxation to guide yourself or others. Find a quiet place so that you can lie down comfortably, with your back on the floor. If you use a head pillow, choose one that is not too high. Relax both arms alongside your body or place them on your belly. Feel your back and the back of your legs on the ground. Entrust yourself to Mother Earth.

Mother Earth will help you to embrace everything, and you do not need to hold on to anything. With your in-breath, be aware of what is. With your out-breath, smile and release whatever thought or feeling is arising.

Now let us use the rays of mindfulness to scan each part of the body, from the top of our head to our toes.

HEAD:

> Breathing in, I am aware of my head—the hair, the skull, the
> brain inside. Breathing out, I smile and release all thoughts
> and feelings that are arising.
> Breathing in, I smile. Breathing out, I release.
> *In, smile. Out, release.*

FACE:

> Breathing in, I am aware of my facial skin and muscles. Breath-
> ing out, I relax my face with a soft smile.
> Breathing in, I smile. Breathing out, I release.
> *Smiling, releasing*

EYES:

Breathing in, I am aware of my two eyes. Breathing out, I smile and relax all the muscles around my eyes.

My dear eyes, I will try to take better care of you. I will allow you to rest more. I will practice looking at things that are beautiful and wholesome, in order to nourish you. Thank you, my dear eyes.

Eyes, resting

MOUTH:

Breathing in, I am aware of my lips and my teeth. Breathing out, I smile.

What great happiness that I can still smile brightly! I promise to speak words of love and kindness. I will practice smiling when there is worry or anxiety in me.

Lips and teeth, smiling

SHOULDERS:

Breathing in, I am aware of my shoulders. Breathing out, I release all the tension and responsibilities to Mother Earth.

I send love and gratitude to my shoulders. I vow to live a gentle, joyful life, so that my shoulders can relax and be more at ease.

Shoulders, relaxing

HANDS:

Breathing in, I am aware of my two hands. Breathing out, I
relax all the muscles and joints in my hands.

How wonderful these hands are that enable me to do so many
things. I can be in touch with the miracles of life, thanks to
them. Thank you, my beloved hands.

Hands, releasing

ARMS:

Breathing in, I am aware of my two arms. Breathing out, I allow
my arms to relax completely.

My arms help me to embrace those who need love and care. I
embrace my own two arms with mindfulness and deep love.

Arms, loving

HEART:

Breathing in, I calm the tension and worries in my heart.
Breathing out, I smile with my heart.

My dear heart, you are so kind and loyal, always there beating
for me. You continue to take care of me so that I may lead
a normal life. Please help me to take better care of you, to
practice putting down my worries, to live more beautifully
and gently. Thank you, my heart, for being so patient and
embracing.

Heart, healing

LUNGS:

Breathing in, I visualize my two lungs—like a giant tree with the trunk dividing into two large branches, and then into smaller and smaller branches. Breathing out, I feel grateful to my lungs for giving me life.

How wonderful that I can breathe in and out so effortlessly! I promise to go outdoors and exercise more often. I also vow to take better care of Mother Earth, because the ocean and the trees are also my heart and lungs.

Lungs, life and freshness

LIVER:

Breathing in, I am aware that my liver is under my rib cage on my right side. Breathing out, I smile tenderly to my liver.

My liver works day and night to filter my blood. Thank you, dear liver, for taking good care of me all these years. I promise to protect you and take better care of you.

Liver, filtering and cleansing

STOMACH AND INTESTINES:

Breathing in, I send my gratitude to my stomach and intestines. Breathing out, I smile and relax my abdominal muscles.

Aware that many illnesses are caused by unmindful consumption, I will try to choose better for my body. I will chew food more slowly and carefully, nourishing my body and mind with positive intention.

Digestion, nourishing

FEET:

> Breathing in, I am aware of my legs, my feet, and my toes.
>
> Breathing out, I send affection and gratitude to them.
>
> What a miracle it is to be able to do innumerable feats each day with these two legs! I vow to take gentle steps upon Mother Earth. Thank you, my dear feet, for being there for me.
>
> *Feet, kissing the Earth*

If there are other parts in your body that have pain or tension, you can use the rest of the time to send extra attention and love to them. Breathe and smile with all your gentleness and friendliness.

You can be aware of the parts in your body that are still healthy and whole, giving rise to gratitude and gladness. This will also give you more strength and energy to nourish and heal the parts that are sick or weakening. Breathe and release the worries and fears that you may be holding in your mind and body. Trust in the capacity of self-healing in your body, and allow it to rest and relax so that it can heal itself.

At the end of the deep relaxation session, you can stretch your body, slowly open your eyes, and smile. "Waking up this morning, I smile. Twenty-four brand-new hours are before me. I vow to live fully and look at all beings with the eyes of compassion."

Maintain this energy of peace, relaxation, and awareness of your body and bring it into the rest of your day. This can bring you deep healing and joy.

Nirvana as Our Daily Business

In Buddhist tradition, we talk about nirvana being the cessation of notions, thoughts, plans, and anxieties. We don't see it as a heavenly place or a mystical state of mind. Thich Nhat Hanh says, "For monastics, nirvana is our daily business," meaning we practice living without excessive thinking and anxiety. We can touch nirvana in our daily life and experience release, letting go, being in oneness with what is, in the moment. We can learn not to keep rehearsing our trauma in the mind, and experience a new freedom from suffering. That is nirvana.

I can attest to the freedom that comes with time and practice. I actually don't think very much about the suffering of my past in my daily life. I just live one moment to the next moment with more peace, more spaciousness. I don't think much about the future. I don't even worry about practical things, such as whether the monasteries will survive the passing away of our beloved teacher. Or, who will take care of me in my old age. I just have full faith and confidence in myself. If I live this moment beautifully, I know the next moment will be beautiful. I live and die beautifully in each moment, so I will live and die beautifully however long I still have on this earth.

Spiritual Practice Is Not about Control

If we have undergone trauma, it is very possible that we approach even beneficial behaviors like eating healthy foods, yoga, exercise, and spiritual practice with a controlling mindset. We want a sense of control and find ways to fix ourselves, to fix the situation, with the premise that we are broken. So we may enter spiritual life with the same habit—being fervent in doing the right thing, obsessive with the practice, striving for higher levels of attainment, and so on.

Look honestly at your practice and see if there is an element of compulsiveness or forcing. That controlling energy will, sooner or later, drive you to exhaustion, frustration, dissatisfaction, and disappointment. You will blame your burnout on the spiritual practice and walk away from it, feeling hopeless and helpless and failing all over again.

Our culture is about always doing something, which gives us a sense of self-worth and value. "I'm always running." How many times have I heard people talk about their stress like this? Yet frantic doing and controlling can impede our healing process. Instead, we can learn to simply sit with what is and listen to it. Listen to our inner child, comforting her, consoling her, "I'm here for you. I listen to you. I want to understand you. I love you."

The Runaway Truck: No Time to Rest

In preparation for the US tour in 2015, my monastery ordered some large trailers for the retreatants to stay in on-site. A few days before the retreat began, two delivery people drove a big truck to drop them off. If you've ever been to Deer Park, you know that the land is full of steep ravines and the roads are narrow, curving, and challenging for large vehicles.

I was standing on the road facing our large lower parking lot when I saw the truck careening toward me. It was rolling downhill on its own without a driver, straight toward the edge of a ravine! A man was running parallel to the truck. He managed to jump up and grab the door on the driver's side, and he vaulted himself into the cab of the truck. The truck ran across the cement road toward the ravine, the driver hauling hard on the steering wheel to try to turn it away from the edge. The head of the truck turned 90 degrees to the right and it stopped, right before it was about to plunge into the ravine! The front wheels were stopped by the raised concrete lip on the side of the road. The truck driver turned off the engine and clambered out of his seat, his face completely bloodless and pale.

It was a traumatic experience for those of us who witnessed it, but it was especially bad for the driver. He immediately called his company. A group of people came to help rescue the truck. It was already after 7 p.m., and they worked until after 11 trying to get the truck out and stabilize it, to bring it back to the company.

I went to bed while they were still working in the dark, and I felt so much compassion for the driver. He had just gone through an extraordinarily challenging experience, but immediately he had to call his company, work together with others to try to rescue the truck, and then deliver the truck back to its proper place. The whole time, most likely he was thinking that he might lose his job, his livelihood, maybe even his house. He would have to fill out a report and face his boss and the consequences the next day. All of this was traumatic, one blow after another. He had no time to sit still to allow his body to relax and his mind to return to his body! All the stress hormones released into his bloodstream did not have a chance to clear out before more were released. When trauma is not properly processed, it is a perfect setup for the development of PTSD.

The runaway truck got me thinking about what would be the best way to deal with similar events in the future. Ideally, right after a potentially traumatic event, someone else should help by taking over the situation. The driver should not have had to make the phone call to his company or to deal with the vehicle after the fact. He should not have had to make decisions or lead activities, so that he could have a chance to step back and let his body adjust to the experience. After the truck had stopped, he should have had a moment to sit down on the sidewalk, and someone should have sat down with him and helped him slow his breathing. He could even have lain down on the ground on his back, getting in touch with the trembling and shaking of his body and relaxing it with mindful in-breaths and out-breaths.

He could guide himself through the process, saying, "It's okay. Everything is okay. The truck stopped, and I am thankful to still be alive." Just thirty minutes like that would allow his body to calm and the earth to absorb all the tension and fear in his body and mind. Someone should have driven him home right after the accident, so he could get in a hot bath to relax or just lie down on his bed, sleep, and then deal with the rest in the morning. Hopefully, his partner would be empathetic and supportive of him, not questioning and blaming him for the accident.

Simple acts like these could help ward off physical and mental illness later in life. To prevent and heal from trauma, sometimes the most valuable element is something we do not have: time to do nothing but heal.

Beyond Duality

My young niece, Sunee, liked the game "Would You Rather" a lot. One time she asked my brother, "Daddy, would you rather eat ice cream that tastes like poop or eat poop that tastes like ice cream?" She insisted on an answer. Finally, my brother replied, "Okay, I'd rather eat poop that tastes like ice-cream." Then Sunee turned to ask me, "What about you, Chô Chô?"* I was forced to make a choice, so I said, "Okay, I'd rather eat ice cream that tastes like poop."

---

* *The actual word for "auntie" in Vietnamese is *cô*, but when my brother, Sonny, tried to teach Sunee to say, "Cô, Cô" for the first time, she looked at his mouth closely and what came out of her own was "Chô Chô." The nickname stuck, and I love it because I am the only "Chô Chô" in the world.

But when I took the opportunity to ask Sunee, "Would you rather eat ice cream that tastes like poop, or poop that tastes like ice cream?" she replied, "Ice cream!" I tried to push her to make a choice, "Which one?" Three times I tried to corner her into a decision. She yelled from the top of her lungs, "Ice cream! Just ice cream!" I turned to my brother and said, "Can you believe it? She would have you eat poop that tastes like ice cream, and me eat ice cream that tastes like poop, but she would be free to eat just ice cream! Wow!"

Think of the choices that we have been forced to make, and the choices that we have imposed upon ourselves. More often than not, they are based in duality, on pairs of opposites, such as good versus bad, you versus me, beauty versus ugliness, coming versus going, and birth versus death. Our mind assigns these values, which then give rise to bodily sensations of desire or aversion, and behaviors of grasping or rejection. In a spiritual life, we learn to examine the extreme polarity of our ideas and perceptions, slowly bringing them to the middle way, known as Right View, when we let go of notions and see reality as it is.

Thich Nhat Hanh has often emphasized the teaching on the Three Doors of Liberation, which are taught in every Buddhist tradition: emptiness, signlessness, and aimlessness. These three profound truths are about interbeing in their essence, and they are our doorways to freedom.

Emptiness, or the teaching of no self. Emptiness does not mean we are nothing or that we do not exist. It just means that who we are is composed of myriad elements; we exist because of the causes and conditions that manifested in time and space; our existence is not disconnected. When we realize we are empty of a separate self, we feel our connection with all things, and we can live with joy and ease. Since nothing has a separate self, everything is connected. This is interbeing.

Signlessness. The form or outer appearance of things—their "sign"—can be deceptive. Water in a cloud looks like a cloud, but then it transforms into rain, and after that the water continues in the plants the rain watered. The form changes, but nothing is ever lost. When we understand the teaching of signlessness—when we are no longer attached to temporary forms—we go beyond conventional ideas about birth and death and enjoy our lives more fully.

Aimlessness. Thich Nhat Hanh pointed out that we are endlessly running after something: love, money, happiness, enlightenment, and so on. Aimlessness means you have no compulsiveness in your goals. You realize you have everything you needed all along. When you understand the teaching of aimlessness, you stop running after things and relax.

The practice of aimlessness in particular can be an antidote to our control issues in ourselves and in our society. Simply enjoy an in-breath as it is. Simply enjoy an out-breath as it is. Enjoy one step at a time. Nowhere to go. Nothing to do. This is it!

Aimlessness leads to pure, unconditional joy. When there's joy, ease, and relaxation in body and mind, the grip for control can also be relaxed and released. Joy is an important element in all the teachings of the Buddha, including the sixteen exercises of mindful breathing, the four immeasurable minds of love, and the seven factors of awakening. (If you wish to learn more about these trainings, please turn to the Selected Resources at the back of this book.) If you are dedicated to the relaxation and enjoyment of what is already available in your body and mind, and can touch moments of gratitude and contentment in your life, you are already practicing to release yourself from the habit of seeking, striving, and controlling.

The ultimate aim in a spiritual practice is letting go, nirvana. Nirvana means the release of the notions of opposites: poop versus ice cream, right versus wrong, relief versus anxiety, my pain versus your pain, reward versus punishment, and even victim versus perpetrator. It is both easy and not easy at all to let go. In tightening our fists and grasping onto thoughts that make us suffer, energy is wasted on tension and pain. In releasing our fists, our hands are wide open, relaxed, and free. Similarly, in releasing and letting go of all notions, we heal our sense of a separate self and become spacious and free.

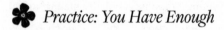 ## Practice: You Have Enough

There is a Buddhist practice called *tri túc* in Vietnamese, meaning "know that you have enough." *Tri* is to know, to remember, to master; *túc* means "enough." Interestingly, *túc* also means "feet." So *tri túc* means that you know and remember that you have enough and take good care of what you have. Additionally, it means you appreciate that you have feet, the foundation of your body!

Our feet symbolize all the conditions of happiness available to us right here and right now. To know that we still have feet is enough to make us happy. Without mindfulness, we take what we have for granted, a destitute on a constant search. We may even take our mindfulness practice for granted, and as a result, we become less fortunate than those who are sincerely seeking a spiritual path and are still full of openness and inspiration.

Knowing that we have enough, we realize that we have everything we ever wish for and that we are enough! This is the true spirit of aimlessness. Awareness of our steps, of our bodily movements, of our in-breaths and out-breaths train us to dwell stably and gratefully in the present moment, which will in turn become a beautiful past, healing the traumas and wounds in our body and mind. It is also the most effective cure for the modern epidemic of restlessness and boredom.

A HAPPY MOMENT

Breathing in and out, I am aware that I'm still alive. I still have myself.

I still have good health conditions. My loved ones are still with me, and my colleagues and friends are surrounding me.

I recognize that this is a happy moment!

Breathing in and out, I recall the image of a person who has loved me and helped me to become more beautiful, more stable, more spacious, more loving toward myself and others.

This is a happy moment!

Breathing in and out, I recall the things someone has thought, done, and said that helped me to be who I am today, and to know what love is.

This is a happy moment!

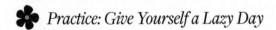 *Practice: Give Yourself a Lazy Day*

In our practice centers, we have a lazy day on Monday every week. Thay had been advised to call it a "rest day" because the idea of laziness has a negative social connotation, but he insisted on keeping this name. Thay once shared that of all the many titles and honors he had received, he enjoyed the title of "Lazy Monk" the most.

To practice being lazy, choose a day in the week or an hour in the day that you can simply be. With the attitude of "nowhere to go and nothing to do," you can enjoy sitting or lying in a hammock, on a rocking chair, underneath a shady tree or, even more lazily, your bed. You may find that being lazy is actually not easy.

Breathe, smile, and relax. Here are some mantras you can say lazily to yourself, to remind yourself you can let go of the habit of doing.

"I can simply be!"

"Thank you!"

"I love you!"

"I am so blessed."

"This is not so bad!"

You can also do what you enjoy most, if that means staying in bed a little longer, reading your favorite book, making a nice breakfast, drinking tea or lemonade, going on a hike—whatever gives you joy. Eat your meals mindfully and lazily, savoring every bite. Keep your lazy day simple with minimal plans and activities, with no goal or anything to strive for. On weekends and on vacation, many of us fill up our itineraries and return from them exhausted. Definitely do enjoy a lazy day, so that you can be truly rested at the end of your free time.

A lazy day or a lazy hour can be enjoyable and replenishing, allowing your mind to be spacious and creative later on when you go back to your tasks. In the true spirit of aimlessness, you can live your life and do what you need to do, but you are actually resting in nirvana. Every moment that your mind rests brightly and peacefully in the here and now, it is a delicious lazy moment, a moment of nirvana.

CHAPTER 6

Concentration as a Strength

The energy of mindfulness carries within it the energy of concentration. When you are aware of something, such as a flower, and can maintain that awareness, we say that you are concentrated on the flower. When your mindfulness becomes powerful, your concentration becomes powerful, and when you are fully concentrated, you have a chance to make a breakthrough, to achieve insight. If you meditate on a cloud, you can get insight into the nature of the cloud.... You can meditate on a person, and if you have enough mindfulness and concentration, you can make a breakthrough and understand the nature of that person. You can meditate on yourself, or your anger, or your fear, or your joy, or your peace.

—THICH NHAT HANH

During our winter holiday retreats, we always invite families to join us in our end-of-year celebrations, and for a couple of weeks our usually quiet monastery becomes a lively place full of rambunctious kids and teenagers. Most families come to spend some quality time with us and each other in nature, unplugged and away from the stresses of work and school, but we also have visitors in search of deeper healing. One year, a fourteen-year-old boy named Kennedy and his mom came for a few days. He asked to have a consultation with me, but once we were sitting together, he was too reticent to speak. I asked him questions until he was finally able to reveal in bits and pieces that he had been sexually abused since the age of five by his father, a drug user. Not until the previous year, when he turned thirteen, had he clearly understood that his father's actions were sexual abuse, and told his mother about it.

Kennedy had handsome features but he looked drained and lost. Poignantly, he asked me, "Is my dad the cause of me not being able to focus in school?" Seeing the expression of distress on his innocent face, I wanted to cry. Adverse childhood experiences (ACEs)* show up in a host of ways, in behaviors that look like attention deficit hyperactivity disorder (ADHD), disturbed sleep, cognitive impairment and memory loss later in life, and general acting out. Child psychologists look for visible signs of stress in children to understand what might have happened to them and how best to intervene. The child may seem distracted or withdrawn. Some kids have nightmares or recurring thoughts of a stressful event or may reenact the trauma in how they play.

Kennedy's mom, Kate, was a single mom. She too grappled with a history of incest in her family of origin. She came to talk to me and shared that early on, she had also suspected something was terribly wrong. She found sores around her son's anus, bruises on his body. He cried out in his sleep. In first grade, Kennedy's schoolteacher informed her that her son had invited his female classmates to sit naked with him in the restroom. Kate instantly recognized that this behavior was not normal for a child and reported to the school counselor and school officials that she was worried about sexual abuse. Unfortunately, they

---

* Adverse childhood experiences, or ACEs, are potentially traumatic events in childhood (0–17 years). They include experiencing violence, abuse, or neglect; witnessing violence at home or in the community; and having a family member attempt or die by suicide. For more on ACEs, see the book by California Surgeon General Nadine Burke-Harris, *The Deepest Well: Healing the Long-Term Effects of Childhood Adversity* (New York: Houghton Mifflin Harcourt, 2018).

dismissed her, saying that she was paranoid and overly suspicious, imagining things because she herself had been sexually abused. As a result, the young mother had to let her son continue to spend time with his father. Then one day when he was eleven, soon after she had dropped her son off at his father's house, the boy called her from a public phone booth, crying.

Kate immediately went to pick him up and reassured him that from then on he would never have to be with his father again. Like many non-offending parents of sexually abused children, she never prosecuted Kennedy's father, probably because she was struggling just trying to make ends meet for herself and her son. Kate tried to make things better for her son. She found a sliding-scale therapist for him to talk to. She brought him to the monastery to practice. She tried so hard to protect her son, but still she was full of regret.

Kate was raising Kennedy alone and was in the process of moving to another state in search of a more positive environment for him, well away from his father. Seeing that they as a family would benefit from some loving support, I urged her to let Kennedy stay at the monastery with us during the summer.

Although she felt ambivalent about leaving Kennedy at the monastery without her, she knew her son desperately needed help. The sisters and brothers were kind enough to allow Kennedy to stay at the monastery free of charge. Kennedy was often quiet, keeping his gaze down, not looking anyone directly in the eyes. When he walked, he tiptoed up on his toes instead of placing the soles of his feet on the ground. His peculiar walk evoked an image of an almost-spent helium balloon bobbing up and down near the ground—his feet only lightly brushing the earth like the dangling string of the balloon.

The first night he was at the monastery without his mother was eventful. As I was about to fall asleep, I suddenly heard a frightening cry. I quickly put on a sweater and went outside, where I saw Kennedy standing there wailing outside the sisters' quarters, his hands gesturing wildly in the darkness. My younger sisters stood aside, bewildered and uncertain of what to do. Immediately I walked up to him and held him tightly in my arms, whispering to him, "It's okay, my dear. Sister D is here with you." That was all I said, and he stopped screaming and wailing. He looked around as if he did not know where or even who he was. I helped him to sit down on the cement floor of the verandah. His legs were stiff and rigid, as if he were paralyzed.

"Breathe, my dear," I said. "Come back to your in-breath and out-breath. You are safe and protected. There is nothing to fear...." Just like that, I was doing guided meditation with him right in front of the nunnery. Gradually, his whole body softened, and he could sit up by himself. A while later, two monastic brothers came along, and Kennedy obediently followed them back to his room in the men's quarters.

Gradually Kennedy overcame his crisis, but he was frequently spaced out, not in touch with his body, or out of control altogether with seizures that had no identifiable basis. Another time I did a guided meditation with him in the main hall, and then I told him to go put on his shoes on the men's side and meet me at the front so we could go for a walk together with the community. After waiting for him a while, he still had not appeared, and I went to investigate. There he was, lying on his back on the floor with his feet waving stiffly in the air while his two hands struggled in vain to put on his shoes. I guessed his body just collapsed on him. He looked at me apologetically.

I froze for a split second and then I burst out affectionately, "You know, you look like a beetle on your back with your legs in the air.

Imagine a cute beetle trying to put on tiny red shoes!" He cracked a crooked smile. I bent down to help him get up and put on his shoes. He leaned on me like a frail old man until his steps became more stable and he was able to walk on his own.

Brain Changes in Trauma

For human beings, the frontal lobe is the most developed part of our brain. In particular, the prefrontal cortex covering the front part of the frontal lobe of the brain is where self-awareness becomes possible. Our animal ancestors are very aware of objects outside of themselves, like a cat who is aware of a mouse, or a mouse of a cat. As humans, we also have the capacity to be aware of our own bodily movements and our own feelings—not just that of the objects outside us.

Scientists have studied the brains of people who have been through traumatic experiences and discovered that brain activity is frequently affected or changed in many areas. MRI scans of the patient's brain show that the frontal lobe, which is responsible for judging, analyzing, and reflecting, will not light up as in a healthy person but instead looks dark. Thus, in trauma, a person suffers not only a psychological injury but also a brain injury. Our ability to focus is impaired. This is why mindfulness practice, which naturally leads to enhanced concentration, is healing for the brain and helps restore our ability to self-reflect.

The Lotus of the Heart

Kennedy shared with me that he often watched pornography online, especially when he was bored, stressed, or depressed. There was a spot, half the size of his fist, between his sternum and his belly button that would contract and spasm violently when he was sexually aroused. He would experience pleasure and pain simultaneously, writhing and doubling over on the floor.

Kennedy had given me a card with a picture he had drawn of a black-and-white lotus blooming in the dark. I told Kennedy to visualize the spot beneath his sternum as the lotus flower he had drawn. He could place his hand on the lotus and breathe with it, sending love and affection to it, visualizing it lighting up and shining. I also advised him to practice being careful about what he would allow his mind to ingest, and to be aware of his daily mindful consumption with his six sense organs, of eyes, ears, nose, mouth, body, and mind.

Sexual abuse is extremely isolating to all involved. The only constant person Kennedy had in his whole life was his mother. Yet one day he hesitantly revealed to me, "Sister D, I don't even trust my own mother. I don't know if she will hurt me, if she will abandon me." That was very painful for him to admit. He felt he couldn't rely on his mother, even though she was making every sacrifice possible to be there and care for him. He was unable to trust her because of the distrust he had for his father and because of the many years that his mother could neither stop the abuse nor protect him.

Staying long-term at the monastery twice over a two-year period, Kennedy slowly opened up to love and joy. He was delighted to learn how to make simple dishes in the monastery kitchen and help out with chores. His ambitions were simple and touching. His eyes lit up when he imagined making breakfast and lunch for himself and his mother. He dreamed of having his own room, where he would have a small corner to sit quietly and drink tea from a cup on which a monastic sister had engraved some loving words for him. His steps became more stable, his gait upright. From a distraught-looking boy, he grew into a stalwart and confident young man.

After he left the monastery, in his subsequent emails to me Kennedy shared about the great progress he had made in school. He enjoyed writing and giving presentations in front of his class and his school. He had good friends, a job, and shared with me excitedly about the process of applying to college. On the way home from work, he loved to stop by a local bookstore and sit in his favorite corner to read.

Kennedy sent me a copy of his college application essay about his experience at the monastery, which I have his permission to share here.

ZEN!

Every morning before sunrise, the monastics and I rose to the ringing of the big bell and the distant chanting of a shrouded sister reverberating across the monastery. Practicing what the monastics termed "noble silence," I would wordlessly switch on the light, don my robes, brush my teeth, and step out from the dorm into the foggy Mississippi night. Streetlamps illuminated my way, casting their reflection on the wet bricks leading to the meditation hall. The same herd of deer that startled me every morning on this journey would bolt from the property into the dark woods. In the warm, pine-scented meditation hall, I would take off my shoes and shuffle in my socks to take my seat among the rows of cushions occupied by monks. We would sit for hours, slowly letting go of our sense of self, paying close attention to each thought as it arose and faded away.

My mornings went like this during my stay at the Zen monastery last year. The simple, compassionate way of life observed by Môc Lan monastics appealed to me on a deep level. It inspired me to take a look at the way that I lived my life and change it for the better. Since my decision to evolve, I've found that I have progressively become more and more like the person that I aspire to be. This evolution, I feel, has helped to prepare me for anything that I might face in life. I am now meditating daily, regulating my thoughts and emotions effectively, and loving myself and others nearly without discrimination. I have over time watched myself become a kind, humble, and gentle spirit who is able to throw himself wholeheartedly into every task, no matter how menial. The greatest happiness that this evolution brings is that it never ceases; I am continually reaching closer and closer to the masterpiece that I want to create of myself.

This evolution is a constant battle. During my second year of high school I was diagnosed with PTSD. The disability, and the seizures that came with it, presented me with a challenge. Either I could let it crush me, as so many others do, or I could find a solution. The search for that solution was what brought me to Môc Lan. The first days there were some of the hardest days of my life, as I had no escape from the memories I had buried for years. Eventually, through discipline and meditative practice, I found that my flashbacks lessened from three times a day to once a month. These results were hard-won, and when I look back at how my life was and how my life is now, I feel a surge of pride in my achievements.

Since my battle for self-improvement has calmed, I am ready to serve as a resource to my community as this college has been for more than a hundred years. I am more than eager to reach my goal of receiving a PhD in conservation biology, which would prepare me for a lifetime of remediating anthropogenic damage to the environment. This college challenges its students to improve, treats them with dignity, and prepares them to enter the workforce, all while serving as a steward of the land on which it was built. I would benefit immensely from an education at this school, as I did from my education at Môc Lan Monastery. I know that the college community would in turn benefit from my admission.

Thank you for your consideration.

In this essay, we can see Kennedy's growth in confidence, stability of mind, and hope for the future. Not only has he healed from his childhood wounds, he has as he puts it, "The greatest happiness that this evolution brings is that it never ceases." Not long ago, Kennedy told me that he is about to graduate from college and is doing very well in life.

Our Unconscious Mind and Our Ability to Focus

The stable atmosphere of the monastery was healing for this deeply traumatized teen boy, just as it had been for me. The basic promise of the path we are exploring with the Five Strengths is that mindfulness leads to concentration, which then gives rise to insights that liberate us from suffering. Concentration as a strength allows us to look deeply into the roots of our consciousness and resolve the suffering buried there. However, many of us with a history of trauma have difficulties with focus and concentration. We get overtaken by negative thoughts in waking life and nightmares when we are asleep. We do not have real rest.

The place where our concentration is most deeply affected is in our store consciousness. Many people report having intense dreams when they are on meditation retreats. Dreams are reflections from our subconscious, which can help us sort, understand, and integrate certain experiences in everyday life, as well as in the past. They are a vision from our subconscious, to help us integrate certain experiences. They can change our relationship with our trauma at the deepest level. The daytime energy of mindfulness manifests in the night, infusing our dreams with awareness, enabling right views, right thinking, and right actions, even when we are asleep. The nighttime energy of healing in turn empowers us in our waking life.

By looking at our dreams, we can access areas that are closed off in our conscious or waking mind and effect changes at the deepest levels. We will find we will sleep better, wake more refreshed, and be better able to focus and utilize our mind for what we wish instead of being carried away by negative thoughts.

Past traumas may cause us to have recurring dreams, with some variations but the same horrifying content. These dreams are telling, reflecting the working of our store consciousness. Unresolved issues, even if they do not manifest in our daily life, will manifest at some point in our dreams. Nightmares and disturbing dreams allow us a view into the depth of our mind, and we can focus on healing them in our daily life, instead of being oblivious to our own suffering and wasting energy on frivolous activities. When there's healing, it also reflects in our dreams, like my dreams about my uncle. He transformed from being an aggressor to a victim and then into a teacher. In my dreams now, I am not just the victim anymore, or simply reacting to the situation blindly, running when someone chases after me. My dreams are radically changed.

In my dreams, I actually find myself making an assessment of the situation, just as I would in waking life. For example, if I see that I am getting lost, I don't panic. I tell myself, *If I go straight, I'll find the way home.* In one dream I was trying to catch up with a group of monastics and feeling lost and abandoned by the group. We were in an open market, full of people and noise and chaos. Suddenly, I paused and told myself, *I don't have to try to get there.* I simply stood still in the middle of the market, and in a moment everything became completely quiet. Everything vanished. There was complete silence and peace, and I woke up with that feeling. In another similar dream, I was in a train station in Japan, with streams of people flowing by during rush hour. It was overwhelming, and I felt utterly lost. Then I thought, *I just need to stop.* I closed my eyes. Everything became quiet. I was standing all alone, secure and calm in myself, in my dream.

Meditation practice and the energy of stopping in our daily life are transmitted to our dreams, so that we become more awake and aware of the situation even while we're asleep—aware of what's happening inside and around us and able to assess what to do and what not to do. As a result, our understanding of the circumstance and thus our reaction to it are changed at the core.

Transforming Trauma in Dreams

I used to have recurring dreams in which I did not know where I was, somebody had abandoned me, or I was trapped in Vietnam. I repeatedly suffered from dreams where I would be chased and pushed down, and made to perform sexual acts with my uncle, cousin, or brother. These disturbing dreams were petrifying and painful to wake up to, and they affected my whole day or even my whole week, often spiraling my mood down into depression or anxiety episodes.

However, as the daily practice of mindfulness shines awareness on all levels of our consciousness including our sleep, through meditating regularly and keeping track of my dreams in my journal, I began to be able to assess my circumstances. Consequently, my habitual reactions of horror and disempowerment would morph in my dreams into new, mindful scenarios.

For more than twenty years, I had horrible, repetitive sexual dreams about my uncle who molested me. Then, one night, I had a different dream. I saw him lying there on the ground, his body emaciated, sickened, with open sores on his skin. Instead of feeling frightened by him, I found a piece of cloth, wet it with water, and dabbed it ever so gently on his wounds to clean them. When I woke up from the dream, I felt a deep, inexplicable tenderness and love in my whole being.

Then, not too long ago, I had another dream. A handsome young man was dressed in a white shirt with a starched collar and long sleeves, his shirt neatly tucked into khaki dress pants. He stood in front of me, and I felt a deep mutual respect and security with this person. I said to him, "Thank you for being my teacher. You have helped me to become who I am." The moment I woke up, I realized that the man had the face of my uncle! It was a huge shock to see him dressing up so fine and gentlemanly as my teacher, but I also had a strong feeling of empowerment and healing.

This is healing at the most basic level of our mind. Your antagonist is no longer a devil or an enemy, but a human being with all their humanness, vulnerability, pain, and even beauty and dignity. You have gained compassion for that person, and you have gained compassion for aspects of yourself that you may have denied for a long time.

Continue to Walk Your Path

The Buddha had a teaching like this: If a negative or frightening thought arises, if you have the capacity to do so, when you're walking, continue to walk with it. If you are sitting, continue to sit with it.

I am so moved by this teaching. It means that we do not try to suppress or forget our scary thoughts. Continue to walk with it in awareness, holding it, embracing it, and calming it. Continue to sit with it, holding it, embracing it, understanding it. In whatever position the body is in, be aware of it and of the feeling that is arising. Of course, you should not force yourself to do this against your better judgement. It's also okay to "change the song" as we explained on page 94.

We can practice looking more objectively at our negative thoughts. *What happened yesterday that might have triggered this mood? Did I have a bad dream? What does this dream mean to me?* It is like you are playing back the video in slow motion. Now that you are awake and watching it, you can see yourself and the situation more clearly. You can think differently, and you can choose to respond differently. Awareness enables you to see possibilities that you have never seen before. Next time a bad mood or dream comes, your mind is prepared to respond differently, in a more mindful, wise, and peaceful way.

I also observe myself throughout the day after a nightmare, recognizing that it makes me more vulnerable, irritable, depressed, and withdrawn. I allow myself a quiet space to hold these feelings tenderly, like I'm being there for the child crying inside of me.

Before I became a nun, after a bad dream I could spiral into depression for the whole day or even week, and it affected every aspect of my life. I would become distant to my partner and my colleagues, lashing out all too easily. Now, I may still have bad dreams, but they are not as frequent or as intense as before. I wake up, I breathe with the dream, I sit with it, I walk with it, and most importantly, I smile to it. If there is some residue, I am able to hold it with equanimity. It does not affect the quality of my day, and that is incredibly empowering.

It is the feeling of helplessness, of powerlessness, that causes us to become despairing, negative, resentful, even vengeful. We may think, *You don't know what pain is. I'll show you what pain is,* and lash out at others. We may become irresponsible toward ourselves and others because people have been irresponsible to us. Thus, we repeat the cycle of abuse, and this is how the victim becomes the perpetrator! Therefore, we need to be empowered with trust and confidence in ourselves, that we are able to be there and take care of what is. We become responsible for ourselves and care for others more appropriately and effectively.

Improving the Quality of Our Sleep

For trauma survivors, healing our dysfunctional sleep patterns is the first step in being refreshed and able to practice mindfulness and concentration in our everyday lives. The best way to take care of our sleep and dreams is by going about our day more mindfully, aware of the triggering factors, such as a haunting thought or a disturbing movie, that may later appear in our dream. What we take in during the day determines our nightly output: the quality of our sleep and the content of our dreams. Immediate input yields not only immediate output but also long-term output, reflected in our worldview, self-perception, thoughts, speech, and bodily actions. As the energy of mindfulness becomes strong in our daily life, the frequency and intensity of our nightmares will diminish.

Bad dreams may also be a result of poor blood circulation from your sleeping posture. The sexual organs, bowels, and bladder are innervated by the same sacral nerves, so if your bowel or bladder are full, signals to the brain can also induce sexual dreams or nightmares. This is why it is helpful to eat your dinner early and keep it light.

In medicine, "sleep hygiene" is prescribed for those who have insomnia or difficult sleep, but it can benefit all of us, especially children and adolescents, and prevent sleep problems later. An hour or so before we go to sleep, we should put aside all electronic gadgets, in order to quiet our mental activity. We can do everything at a more leisurely pace, take a shower, and sit quietly for a few minutes. If we have a habit of reading before bed, then we should choose something peaceful and light. Reading from an actual book may be better than from an electronic gadget, since the device's light may be stimulating to the brain, keeping us from falling asleep.

In our bedroom, we should not work or keep anything that is associated with work. Turn off all the lights and all our electronic devices. Light from computers and electronics can interfere with our brain waves and disturb our sleep. Keep the room completely dark. As you lie down in bed, practice body scanning and deep relaxation (see chapter 5, page 107 for practice instructions), sending love and gratitude to your body.

It is important to have a regular sleeping schedule and to go to sleep early enough that your body has time to rest and replenish itself. Many people report they have the most restful sleep of their life when they come to a monastery—simply because it's the first time since they were children that they've tried to regulate their sleep! Going to sleep by 9 or 10 p.m. and waking up early is healthier, more in accordance with the circadian rhythm, and thus more beneficial than going to sleep at midnight and waking up late in the day.

As I lie on my bed at night, I often think that if I were to not wake up from this night, I would have nothing to regret. I have done my best to live my life kindly, so I can leave anytime, with peace in my heart. One evening, as I was midway through writing this book, I swallowed something that might have accidentally had a fine piece of metal in it.

In the dark of the night, I thought of the possible consequences, such as gastric bleeding. I breathed and did a review of my life, experiencing no feeling of regret. *Of course, this book would be unfinished if I were to die this very night,* I thought, *but the preliminary manuscript was already out there, and Hisae, my editor, would take good care of it.* That was the only thing that came to my mind. Then I drifted into a peaceful sleep. Waking up the next day, my first thought was *I am still alive! I guess I'm okay.* I breathed, smiled, and sent gratitude to my body for giving me another day to live.

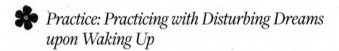

Practice: Practicing with Disturbing Dreams upon Waking Up

If you wake up suddenly in the middle of a nightmare, do not go back to sleep right away. Simply breathe and relax your body.

> *Breathing in, I am aware that I just had a nightmare.*
> *Breathing out, it is okay. It was only a dream.*

Follow your breath until your heart beats slower, and your breathing calms. Go wash your face and empty your bowel and bladder, which will help prevent the dream from returning and causing you further distress.

Practice: Reflecting on the Contents of Your Dream

When you wake up from a disturbing dream, you may want to lie in bed for a while, returning to your mindful breathing and relaxing your body, part by part. Later, when you are more fully awake, you can bring up the contents of your dream in your sitting meditation so that you have a deeper understanding of the unresolved issue in your store consciousness.

Relaxing and anchoring yourself in your breath, try to identify the triggering factors and how they may be affecting you. Visualize how you may think, speak, and respond to the situation differently, with more awareness, clarity, and autonomy. This will develop your capacity to be proactive, instead of habitually falling into the role of a passive victim. Whether you are involved in the dream as a victim or a perpetrator, these practices can help you understand yourself better, regulate your emotions, and transform certain habits and situations in your life.

You can also keep a journal about your dreams to observe your own transformation and healing over time.

🌸 Practice: Keep a Dream Journal

We dream at least four to six times a night. Yet, most of us do not remember our dreams, and if we do, those dreams are usually very intense or toward the morning, close to waking. Since dreams can reflect the contents of our subconsciousness, including the unresolved issues, it can be beneficial to keep a dream journal to gain insights into them.

You can jot down your dream when you first wake up and/or write about it in greater detail later in the day. Write from your stream of consciousness, allowing thoughts and feelings and images to flow out naturally from your mind, without censorship or concerns for structure or quality.

Make time to sit with the dreams that you feel are important and revealing to you. Afterward, you can write in your dream journal your insights and discoveries about the significance of your dreams.

Note how the nature and content of your dreams as well as your view and responses may change over time as you practice mindfulness and self-love.

CHAPTER 7

Insight as a Strength

With the powerful energy of concentration, you can make a breakthrough and develop insight. It's like a magnifying glass concentrating the light of the sun. If you put the point of concentrated light on a piece of paper, it will burn. Similarly, when your mindfulness and concentration are powerful, your insight will liberate you from fear, anger, and despair, and bring you true joy, true peace, and true happiness.

—THICH NHAT HANH

I received a few beans as a gift about ten years ago, and they have become the most powerful Dharma instruments for me. They are an heirloom variety of beans known as orca beans or yin-yang beans: one half of the dried bean is pure white, the other shiny black. In the white half there is a black dot, and in the black half there is a white dot, just like in a yin-yang sign. *In this, there is that, and in that, there is this.* They illustrate the profound teaching of interbeing perfectly. So, I have humorously called them "Interbeans." Brian, a dear practitioner friend creatively collaged black and white beans to make a giant model of an Interbean for me, so now when I give a talk I can hold it up and even those in the very back of the hall can see it.

The interbeing between trauma and healing—that each contains elements of its opposite—is one insight on the path of transformation, which takes some practice to gain. Another insight is the awareness of trauma in families: transgenerational or intergenerational trauma. While the handing on of trauma over generations is now becoming accepted through the study of epigenetics, what is less well understood is that our healing in the present can also transform our ancestral trauma.

My mother had been sexually abused as a teenager, and then I was sexually abused as a child. Through the work I do today, I see my mother very differently from how I saw her in the past. I shared the story of my mother in my first book, *Healing: A Woman's Journey from Doctor to Nun*. She came from a poor family in the arid province of Quang Ngai. At fifteen, she went alone to the big city of Saigon to look for work in order to help her mother, my beloved grandma, feed the rest of her family. My mother was not educated, and she first worked as a servant. According to my grandmother, her employer attacked her. Each night, the man she worked for would come to her little corner where she slept at the back of the house. She would curl up under her bamboo bed, but he would not let her be. He used a broom to poke her and get her out from under the bed. Broken in body and spirit, she wandered the streets. Her education was minimal, she had no skills, and she ended up sleeping with American soldiers for cash. What else could a poor, uneducated girl do? What could all the peasant girls do in a city in the midst of a raging war? No war promotes honest living. Thay once said to me, "What happened to your mother also happened to the whole country."

Transgenerational Trauma and Interbeing

Interbeing, as symbolized by our Interbean, is a critical tool for understanding and healing our pain. Modern medicine now has a more holistic understanding of trauma than in the early days of psychology, when the term "shell shock" was coined in Europe during World War II. In the 1970s the designation of post-traumatic stress disorder, or PTSD, was created in the United States to apply to the many military veterans returning from Vietnam, deeply scarred by what they had seen and done. Trauma was seen then as an individual matter, as if somehow it was normal to be untraumatized by the horrors of war, and these veterans were just unfortunate or weak. Now we see how untrue and unwholesome this view is.

When we are not aware of ourselves, when we are checked out, trauma can accumulate not only in ourselves, but in our entire family, and eventually our community, and even our country. The medical community now also talks about collective trauma that endures over centuries, such as the trauma from slavery in the United States; acute national trauma, such as when a country experiences a cataclysmic event like 9/11; or even global trauma, such as the trauma caused by what is happening to our planet due to climate change, and most recently, the COVID-19 pandemic. We also recognize transgenerational trauma, which is passed on from one generation to the next.

When we apply Buddhist psychology and the insight of interbeing to trauma, we gain a radical understanding of suffering. With the eyes of a Buddha, we see that in a flower there are non-flower elements such as water, soil, sunshine, the gardener's hands, the florist's expertise—all are present in the flower. If any one of these elements were to vanish, the flower would also not exist. *This is because that is. This is not because that is not.* In this, there is that, and in that there is this. In the one, there is the all.

This insight is revelatory and easy to comprehend when we talk about pleasant phenomena such as flowers, but more difficult to accept and embrace when we talk about unpleasant things. By acceptance, by the way, I do not mean we accept or excuse the actions of those who have traumatized us. I simply mean that we recognize that both perpetrator and victim are caught in a self-reinforcing cycle of trauma and abuse that goes back generations, and indeed, may be more ancient than the human race itself. The insight of interbeing between perpetrator and victim can liberate us from hostility, shame, and a host of other negative mental formations.

Through my practice, I have come to understand that my uncle and I inter-are. The people of Vietnam were collectively traumatized by being colonized by the French, then by war with the Americans. As a runaway teen and then a soldier during the war, my uncle was traumatized, and then he passed trauma on to me. Just as we can see the relationship between individual and collective suffering, we can also see the interrelationship between this pain and our aspiration to understand and heal suffering for ourselves and others. Our pain and our liberation inter-are. Radiant flowers do not grow on marble. They grow from the dirt. It cannot be any other way.

For me, the teaching of interbeing is both profound and practical. It encompasses everything that we refer to as nondiscrimination, equanimity, and letting go. If we reach a level of practice where we can see how even our most painful experiences are part of who we are, and we can cherish all of who we are, then we are applying the teaching of interbeing in our daily life. We are living the teaching. This "right view" helps us to develop our insight into the nature of interconnectedness, which in turn fosters true love, opening the path of love for ourselves and others. True love in this light—one of the mindfulness trainings we will explore in part 3—allows us to see that your happiness is also my happiness and, similarly, your suffering is also mine.

Why is this work of healing so important? We wish the trauma to end with us, and we want to transform our pain into understanding and compassion. In interbeing, the individual is in the collective, and the collective is in the individual. Everything will manifest from the subconscious to the conscious levels of the individual and of the collective, what we Buddhists call the store consciousness and the mind consciousness. They are not one, but neither are they two, nor are they separable. Whatever is overwhelming, unspeakable, unacceptable, and untransformed by us will be transmitted to the next generation. Whatever we cannot transform, we will transmit. We will transmit it to our children, our grandchildren, our spouses, our friends. We will transmit it through our energy, our words, our bodily reactions, and our thoughts. In daily life, our loved ones and those close to us observe our actions, hear our words, and they can suffer from our thoughts. In fact, they absorb all of it.

Therefore, time alone does not heal; the passage of time can bring more sadness, pain, anger, resentment, and destructive behaviors. Time can amplify trauma, and it can echo over generations in a family, in a community, and in a nation.

To face that abuse, that pain, that sadness is to transform it so that it is not passed on to the next generations. This is transgenerational liberation from trauma.

Mindfulness enables us to be in tune with our body and mind in the present moment. True to the insight of interbeing, in the present, there is the past, and there is the future. We cannot change the past. Whatever happened has already happened. Yet by taking good care of the present moment we are taking care of the past. We are healing ourselves and our ancestors. Whatever we do transform, we also transmit. Thus, in transforming and healing our trauma, we are also

taking care of our future generations, preventing the cycle of transgenerational trauma.

Legacies of Childhood Sexual Trauma

We have been told that, anatomically, the body renews itself continually, giving us a brand-new body every seven years. The cells in our
body continually die and regenerate throughout our lives. Why then do
people who have experienced childhood abuse continue to feel the pain
as intensely as if it had just happened yesterday, or as if it is still happening, even after they grow up? It is because of the way our mind works.
Our bodies may have renewed themselves, but the way we view our
bodies is still the same, and the way we recall the traumatic experience
is the same. Our attitude about ourselves—now, as adults—is largely
unchanged from when we were children. The unwholesome energies
of the perpetrator are still viscerally alive in us.

Focusing on the area of family trauma, we can see vicious cycles of
transgenerational trauma frequently happening two generations in a
row, and sometimes three generations or more. My mother had been
sexually abused, and I was sexually abused. At a conference in Vietnam
where I spoke about the issue of transgenerational sexual abuse, two
sisters came up to me afterward and told me that this was exactly what
had happened in their family. Their grandmother had been sexually
abused, then their mother was sexually abused, and then they were sexually abused. They had all suffered from incest, and the sisters wanted
to find a way out.

I was deeply moved by their coming forward to speak with me.
The act of speaking and being heard—the practice of loving speech
and deep listening, which we will explore in part 3—is healing for both

the speaker and the listener. We hugged each other and they expressed their aspiration to transform the suffering of the family so that it would end with them and not be transmitted to their children.

As we discussed in chapter 3, "Trust as a Strength," many people who experience sexual abuse as children or as teenagers end up having dysfunctional relationships and unstable families as adults. Through the power of affinity, when you are not stable you may attract or be attracted to someone else who is not stable. For example, a young woman may be drawn to an alcoholic or an abuser like her own father, for several reasons. One is that this is what love looks like to that person. Another is that the psyche attempts to understand and resolve its traumas by working its way through situations that have similarities to the past. In this way, an already traumatized person brings further harm upon themselves and their children.

I met a young woman whose mother, a survivor herself, had gone through many relationships. This young woman said that when she was a girl her mother was always at work, but the boyfriends, one after another, stayed home and molested her from the age of seven. The mother did not detect the symptoms and signs of abuse even though the little girl became depressed, was afraid to stay home with the boy-friends, and developed angry outbursts and temper tantrums. Many children of parents who have suffered from sexual abuse will also experience it themselves, often because their mothers and fathers do not know how to take care of their own painful feelings, so they are not present enough to recognize or confront what is going on with their children. They may not be available physically, emotionally, or mentally to take care of their children.

Looking more deeply, while we can provide our children with material things like clothes, cars, electronics, and so on, we should not forget or fail to understand that what our children may need most is our presence. As we have seen from the story of Claire in chapter 3 on trust, the potential psychological impacts of our physical or emotional absence can be devastating.

Hurt People Hurt People

A person may not be conscious of a trauma they experienced in the past. The memory of the trauma remains latent in their store consciousness, untransformed. Whatever past mistreatment or abuse they endured might have caused injuries to their awareness and cognition, and their capacity for compassion and empathy. Through unconscious negative thoughts, actions, and speech, they may rehearse their trauma in their store consciousness which, at some point, will manifest into their mind consciousness as abusive and harmful thoughts, speech, and behaviors. Thus, the victim may perpetrate the exact same abuses they themselves endured earlier.

When we are not aware of what is going on inside of us and around us, we are at risk of getting hurt and hurting others. In this way the trauma may continue to surface; someone who has experienced trauma may become susceptible to post-traumatic stress and further victimization.

When we are lost in deep pain, despair, or confusion, we become engulfed in the past and not aware of what is going on around us. Entrenched in multitudinous emotions, overwhelmed by pain, confusion, and sorrow, we may not be alert to what is happening. We might end up in the wrong place at the wrong time, therefore putting ourselves in dangerous situations. Or we may be hypervigilant and on guard but still not in touch with our present reality.

And then, in turn, we may become the one who causes new trauma to others. This points to a poignant relationship that most of us are not aware of: that the perpetrator is at the same time the victim. The victim and the perpetrator inter-are. Whatever the mind most frequently rehearses, it will manifest in thoughts, speech, and bodily actions. A victim of sexual abuse may be haunted by the traumatic experience, which may in turn push him or her to reanimate the trauma for relief, either by seeking pornography or sexual contact. At some point, we may force sex on someone else the way it was forced on us. If we are in danger of becoming the perpetrator, it is vital for us to learn to love and forgive ourselves first and foremost, to prevent passing on harm to others. Once we can embrace ourselves, we then know how to take care of our own suffering, and we can take care of the suffering that might have been revolving around our loved ones for so long.

I hope that this book can be helpful to all who have encountered trauma, in whatever role. Primarily I write for the survivors of trauma, but witnesses and perpetrators of the same actions are not unscathed. I do not see perpetrators as demons or irredeemable. Because as humans we are all interconnected, with mirror neuron structures in our brains that depend upon social interaction for our growth and healing, we all undergo suffering and experience it viscerally and mentally, whatever our roles may be in a situation. Moreover, I recognize that given certain conditions every one of us is capable of being a perpetrator, a transmitter of suffering to ourselves and others, if we do not know how to care for our mind and mental states of greed, craving, anger, revenge, ignorance, despair, and jealousy.

Hopefully, from these insights of interbeing, we can practice to forgive ourselves and feel inspired to practice healing for others whose lives we may have affected with our actions or inactions. Deep down, no one is programmed to want to hurt others. Even psychopaths and those with certain organic brain diseases that cause them to be ruthless and impervious to people's pain and suffering are also victims of their own neurological and mental illnesses. For most perpetrators, it usually goes back to their childhood, where there was almost always abuse—sexual, physical, verbal, or mental. We cause others suffering because we have suffered ourselves. When we understand that hurt people hurt people, another dimension of deep healing opens up for us.

Will's Story

In 2016, I helped facilitate a retreat for young adults at Deer Park Monastery. A young man named Will arrived a day late, and he brought with him a gigantic iguana. It would crawl all over Will's upper body, and he stroked it affectionately, making its scaly body seem softer. Will did not interact with the people around him, but he would often look at the iguana eye-to-eye as it perched on him. The iguana was Will's only friend.

The next morning, I saw Will standing alone in a corner of the meditation hall and looking distressed. I put my hand on his shoulder and whispered to him, "How are you doing?" He looked at me, suspicious and frightened, but then out of desperation he said to me, "Sister, can I talk to you, please?" I sensed that this young man was suffering deeply, so I told him to walk outside with me. Will opened his heart and shared with me his story.

About four years ago, a young man whom Will had met recently called him and asked if he wanted to go out with him and his friends. Will was home alone that day, bored and restless, so he decided to join them. They drove him to a deserted alley in the city and told him to cover his face with a nylon stocking as they had. Then they attacked a young man who happened to be walking by. They kicked him, they beat him ruthlessly, and then they ran away—except for Will, who bent down to check whether the victim was still breathing or not. In that moment, Will saw the young man's face, and that he was still breathing.

Will left the scene and came home, but he could not forget the young man's face. Haunted, he kept checking the police reports in the newspapers to see if there was any news about somebody being beaten, hospitalized, or killed from that incident. There was no such news, so he felt assured that the young man was somehow okay.

Yet, Will could not be okay from then on. His sense of normalcy began to unravel. He worked as a chef, but after that incident, he became afraid of himself, troubled by the irrational thought that he might poison people someday if he cracked with crazy thinking. He eventually lost his job in that restaurant. Then he tried to find another job in which he could work all by himself at night, so he wouldn't have to interact with people. He couldn't concentrate on the new job either, so he lost that job too. He ended up staying in the basement of his parents' house for almost four years. He didn't have contact with anybody. Then his sister talked to him about going to the retreat for young adults and begged him to come to it. He reluctantly went to the retreat, with a glimmer of hope that he might be able to heal himself from the trauma he had been experiencing the last four years.

Will told me that he checked in the retreat very late the night before. When he finally went to his assigned spot in the monastery dorm, he suddenly caught sight of a young man who looked exactly like the person he and his friends had assaulted four years ago. Even though this person at the retreat was of a different ethnicity, something about his face reminded Will of the victim, and he freaked out. He ran out of the room and stayed in his car the whole night. He could not be in the same room with that person. He was still shaken up in the morning and desperately wanted to talk to me.

Will told me, "Now I am reliving the whole experience!" In the peaceful surroundings of the monastery, his traumatic memories of the event came back full force.

Interbeing between the Perpetrator and the Victim

We can contemplate on interbeing to understand the intimate connection between the perpetrator of a trauma-generating crime and his victim. In Will's case, even though he was both a witness and a perpetrator of a violent assault and he had escaped safely from the scene, the victim's face was etched in his mind. The suffering of that unknown young man became the suffering of Will. Somebody's suffering becomes your suffering, and your suffering becomes somebody else's suffering. We carry on each other's experiences and emotions. Time and space cannot remove us from one another.

Will relived his trauma as he recounted his story to me. It was intensely upsetting for me to listen to his story and to witness the suffering so alive in his contorted face and trembling body. I suggested to him that we would take a short break. I went to the washroom to wash my face. I did walking meditation on my way to the washroom—one step with one breath at a time. When there is a strong emotion or when I am not sure of what to do next, walking meditation can calm my mind and relax my body. Relaxation, calmness, and spaciousness foster clarity and understanding. While I was in the washroom, an insight and a possible course of action came to me.

Will was still sitting there, with his hands covering his bent head. He looked somewhat relieved to see me coming back. I quietly asked him, "Would you like to talk to this young man? Would you like to say sorry to him?" Will looked at me with his eyes wide opened. He panicked, "No, I can't do that!" I gently persisted, "Well, think about it, my dear. This is your chance." We sat in silence for a while. Then he said, "Okay. Can you help me?"

It was time for breakfast, so I had to wait for Will's roommate, the other young man, to finish his breakfast before I could talk to him about Will. I got some food for myself, but Will was too anxious to eat breakfast. He just sat there, his hands tapping on his knees nervously and his legs jerking in constant restless motions. After eating, I went to talk to the young man who looked like the assault victim to Will. I had met Andy in the previous retreats and had established a strong rapport with him, so I was able to approach him easily about this difficult task. I told Andy about Will's story and added, "Can you be so kind as to sit there for Will, so that he can share his pain and his suffering, and he can say that he is sorry? He needs to be able to express his remorse." Andy was well aware of the truth and reconciliation practice we have in the monastery called Beginning Anew. He responded empathetically, "Sure, Sister D. I can do that."

I invited the two young men to sit face-to-face. Will could not look at Andy's face at first. Instead, he kept looking down at the ground and fidgeting his hands and squirming in his seat. I briefly summarized the assault incident to Andy right in front of Will and then added that Will had been traumatized and suffering tremendously ever since. Then I said to Will, "Andy is very kind to be here for you, so you can say whatever you wish to say to him."

Immediately Will said, "I'm sorry, man. I didn't mean it. I didn't want to hurt you. I'm really sorry." Even though Andy only bore a faint resemblance to the victim, Will still talked to him as if he were the actual victim of his violent crime. He was crying as he added, "I didn't know what I was doing. You know, I've been suffering these last four years. Please forgive me. Please forgive me." His entire body was trembling.

Andy listened deeply. He leaned forward to be closer to Will. He said gently, "It's okay. It's okay. It's okay. I forgive you." At one point their knees touched, because they were sitting so close. Will kept leaning in, and Andy put his hands on Will's knees and said, "It's okay. I forgive you. Just take care of yourself. Don't hurt yourself. Don't hurt other people anymore."

They sat quietly with each other for a while. Then I suggested that they hug each other, and they did. I placed my hands on their shoulders and guided them through the hugging meditation, "Follow your in-breaths and out-breaths.... Give rise to gratitude that you are here for each other. Know that you are not outside of each other. Your happiness is his happiness. His suffering is your suffering. Forgive yourself so that you have the energy to go forward in your life. Take good care of yourself, and the victim inside you...."

Will and Andy remained still in each other's embrace. Afterward, they patted each other on the shoulder. Will was visibly more relaxed. He smiled and his shoulders dropped down loosely. It was like they were two long-lost brothers, now united. I said to them, "Can you stay in touch with one another?" Smiling, they exchanged their phone numbers and their emails. When I saw Andy at another retreat this year, I asked Andy about Will. Andy said that they continued to stay in touch, and Will has been able to get a job and is doing so much better. Through speaking and being heard in the safe container of the conversation at our monastery, Will was able to begin his life anew.

Patrick's Story: A Vietnam Veteran

Patrick D. was a Vietnam veteran who came to one of our New York retreats in 2016. He told us that he was homeless, but he was neatly dressed and wiry and healthy of body, riding his bicycle every day to attend the retreat activities. He was quiet and reserved the first two days. I noticed that every time he sat down on the ground, he always took something out of his bag and placed it in front of him.

As Patrick became more at ease in the group, he opened up and shared eloquently about his experience in Vietnam. He had been suffering from post-traumatic stress since the time he came back from Vietnam, which was then more than forty years ago. The image of his comrades blown to pieces in front of him continued to haunt him in his daily life. He had written this experience down in an article that he shared with me:

> Every single dead soul of every single casualty—soldier
> and civilian alike—from that stinking, rotten, un-winnable
> war just showed up inside that place and elbowed their way
> inside me without even asking my permission, and then they
> made themselves right at home for the next forty goddamn
> years, right up until this very moment ... They decided to
> hitchhike ... to turn me into a human [expletive] hearse—or
> better yet, a living, breathing, haunted house, a body bag ...
> I've been carrying around all those poor wandering bastards
> inside me, free of charge, ever since.

To aid his own healing, Patrick started to carry around with him a handmade wooden statue of a Vietnamese farmer bending down to plant rice. This was the object that he always reached out of his bag and placed in front of him whenever he sat down. He said it helped him to calm the fear and hatred that would rise up in him, day and night.

One day, as we were gathered for a Dharma sharing circle, he burst out, "Seeing my so-called enemy, the Viet Cong, was only about four feet tall and planted rice or made crude wooden coffins for a living and were way poorer than any of my Irish immigrant relatives or me ever were ..." He broke down and cried.

All of us in who were present started crying while listening to him share his story. A Vietnamese nun, Sister Eternity, spontaneously stood up, walked toward him and opened her arms to embrace him in front of everyone. It was a moment of healing for everyone in the room. Patrick could finally make peace with the VCs, the Vietnamese people, and his memory of the war in the presence and the embrace of our Vietnamese monastic Brothers and Sisters.

Before he left, Patrick gifted me a mask that he made with a drawing of a soldier holding a gun in one hand and a baby in the other, and on the inside of the mask, he wrote, "For Doctor-Sister Dang Nghiem. You Healed MY BROKEN HEART."

Patrick's healing was my own too, since I never knew my father, also an American GI according to my grandmother. Patrick could have been my biological father for all I knew. If my own father is still alive and out there, I hope that he can experience the sense of reconciliation and peace that eventually came to Patrick.

But then, I also know that my father can experience it in me.

Just Mercy

Somebody once wrote to me that when I share about my feeling of compassion for perpetrators of brutal crimes, they worry people may think that I'm condoning the abuse and the abusers.

Please allow me to pose a question. *For those of us who have held on to the resentment and pain of being the victim of abuse for a long time, how has that helped us heal?* The perpetrators have been unjust, cruel, and inhuman toward us at a point or points in time, but they have since left our lives. They may have died or are long gone. Yet, we may faithfully continue to mistreat our own body and mind. We might let our life be shadowed by the past instead of living the present moment. Ultimately, we need to give mercy and forgiveness to ourselves, for perpetuating the impact of abuse.

Forgiveness is not a kind of amnesia, a forgetting of the past. As long as our mind is intact, we will remember our past experiences. Only understanding and compassion can liberate us from our abusers. They are not outside of us. They are in us, in every cell of our bodies. They are intricately, inexplicably a part of us. We cannot remove them from our memory, but we can transform our memory. They are us and we are them. The insight of interbeing—"this is in that," "this is because that is," and "this *is* that"—ultimately leads us to forgiveness, freedom, and liberation.

After I contracted Lyme disease, my abnormal urinary frequency—one of the symptoms resulting from my childhood sexual trauma—worsened. At my lowest point, every night I woke up five to seven times to use the restroom, and the amount of urine was copious. My sleep was, needless to say, very disturbed. I felt as if everything vital in my body were draining out of my body, down to my bone marrow, and every drop of energy was also draining out of me. One night, as I was wobbling my way to the restroom again, probably for the seventh time, a thought arose in my mind: *If my uncle had known I would continue to suffer this much after more than thirty years, he would not have abused me.* That thought, in the middle of the night, infused me with an unknown sense of peace and softness. *If he had known that I would suffer this much, for this long, he would not have done it.* I had never thought of my uncle in this light, but thanks to the practice, I could now see the possibility of his being different from the monster I had made of him in my mind. I could see him as a human being. I could see him as a victim of his ignorance, of his own abuse, of his own confusion. This line of thinking was unexpectedly liberating for me.

In his book *Just Mercy*, lawyer Bryan Stevenson gives accounts of convicts on death row or in lifetime imprisonment, and the horrifying acts they have done or sometimes were falsely accused to have done. He also shared about their battered childhoods. He asserts, "Mercy is when you give to those who are undeserving, who are un-expecting it." That is true mercy. Who among us is undeserving? You may disagree, but as a Buddhist nun, I have seen over and over again that we all deserve mercy. We all deserve forgiveness. First and foremost we forgive ourselves, and it is from that very space that we are able to care for ourselves and others. Instead of believing that the perpetrators are outside of us, deserving only punishment, we recognize that we can help take care of one other, so that all can heal.

Somebody may abuse us, abandon us, or betray us with their words or bodily actions, but we must make sure that we do not abuse, abandon, or betray ourselves with our thoughts, words, and deeds. If we can do that for ourselves, then we will no longer suffer from abuse, abandonment, or betrayal. Our hearts may sink for a moment, but we deserve to be able to breathe, smile, and move on to live as fully as we can.

To attend to our inner child, to live the present moment, to understand the ordeal that we all must have gone through, is to gain understanding, compassion, and forgiveness and thus achieving liberation from past trauma and suffering. We reclaim our sovereignty to the time and the treasures we still have on this earth. We apply our energy to live beautifully and to help others by sharing concrete teachings and practices so that they, too, can heal. Only in this way can we truly help minimize the abuse in the world and nurture deep healing. It is only from a place of healing that our service is most empowering.

In Vietnamese, we have the word *ân hận,* meaning "to regret something." We may regret something that we did or said that hurt other people. We may regret something about our life, for being poor, for having the parents we had, or having married that person, or for being in an abusive relationship, etc. In the word *ân hận, ân* means "gratitude" and *hận* means "resentment." There is such wisdom embedded in language! When we experience regret, we do have two options: one is to become resentful; the other is to become grateful.

Resentment may add to the energy of pain, confusion, anger, and hatred in us, which may cause us to waste our life energy and, in the extreme, drive us to become abusers ourselves. If we can practice mindfulness and heal, we may actually feel a sense of gratitude for what we have gone through. Many people who come through their traumas with a sense of healing report feelings similar to mine.

> *I am who I am today because of all the experiences I have gone through in my life, including many physical, verbal, and sexual traumas. It is because of these experiences and because of the transformation and healing I have found through the practice that I have been able to help many people heal and transform. In the face of all the abuse and trauma I experienced in life, I am no*

longer saddened or swept away by my past. I can speak about the
trauma with peace and stability and clearly see a way out.

Suffering Is Nonpersonal

When we think about trauma or about situations of injustice, we usually identify with the victims. We think, "*He* did that to me. *She* said that to me. *They* took it away from me. *They* hurt me."

The truth is that we all have also hurt other people. A lot of the time we cause hurt and pain without even knowing why, because we may not think about the event deeply and thoroughly. We were reactive, driven by anger and frustration to harsh speech and cruel behaviors. This could be because we had been victims of cruelty at some point in our childhood, teenage years, or adult years. We may not relate these incidences from the past to the present situation, but they are all related to each other, the way one wave may serve as the foundation and momentum for another wave, accumulating and building up on one another to form larger waves and even tsunamis. The suffering of our parents, ancestors, other people, and other living beings have also become our own suffering; all are deeply enmeshed and intertwined. The countless waves of suffering are immense, persisting through space and time. While the sufferers may have become faceless and nameless over time, the suffering remains real and surges forward into the present.

Beginning Anew

Thanks to the practice of Beginning Anew, Will had a chance to begin to heal and move on with his life. All of us can practice Beginning Anew, regardless of our circumstances. We don't have to be abusers to benefit greatly from this powerful practice.

Beginning Anew has four steps or parts, and true to the teaching of interbeing, if you practice one part, you are practicing the other three. In our retreats, we always hold Beginning Anew with a partner, but you can also adapt the basic process of expressing your hurts and regrets to yourself.

1. Hello and thank you—watering the flowers. We greet ourselves or our partner and express our appreciation, selecting the flowers of their good qualities to water in them.

2. I'm sorry—expressing regrets. We express regrets for anything we have done to hurt ourselves or others.

3. It hurts—expressing hurts. We express ways in which others have hurt us.

4. Resolution—finding a way out. We propose and commit to practices that can help us not to repeat our unskillful actions or speech. We express gratitude and bring the practice to a close.

1. Hello and Thank You

In the first part, we say "hello" and "thank you" to all that is. We "water the flowers" of the aspects of ourselves we wish to cultivate and grow. We recognize we are capable of everything. We are capable of acts of beauty and also ugliness. Everything is in us. There is nothing to reject and nothing to hold on to. Yet, our built-in tendency is to be swept away by the negativity in ourselves and in our life, and to be neglectful of all the wonders available to us. Therefore, it is essential that we consciously recognize and acknowledge the beauties and the blessings that we still have. The practice of mindful breathing enables us to stop and look deeply into our life as it is in the present moment.

The nineteenth-century French psychologist Pierre Janet said, "Traumatic stress is an illness of not being able to be fully alive in the present." The truth is that most of us are not able to be fully present and fully alive in the present moment. Thus, it is an invaluable help to be able to recognize that, "This is an in-breath. This is an out-breath" and to rest in the breath, "Breathing in, I am aware that I am still alive. Breathing out, I smile to life." Or we can affectionately say, "Hello dear me. I know I am still here, and I am thankful."

For those of us who suffer from traumas, the sheer fact of being alive and following our breathing may be extremely difficult and painful. We may feel triggered and suffocated if we try to anchor our mind in the present moment and in our breathing. Consequently, the practice of mindful breathing is a practice of love and patience with ourselves, one moment and one breath at a time. Slowly, we train ourselves to come back to our breath and to be okay with it and to accept it as it is. This, in turn, trains us to be able to be with what is, with what was, with what will be, and to be okay with it all. To embrace it as it is and not try to manipulate it, run away from it, or become drowned in it. Of course, if it is extremely triggering to follow the breath, we can practice being aware of our steps, our hands, or of a part of our body that is more neutral or safe to us. We can come back to the practice of mindful breathing later when we feel more stable in our body and mind.

2. *I Am Sorry*

The second part of Beginning Anew is expressing our regrets. It also means to say, "I'm sorry" to ourselves and for what we have put ourselves through. In Will's case, he had imposed the pain and the suffering on another person, then the pain and suffering of that person became his. The perpetrator has become the victim, and if the victim does not know how to take care of his or her own trauma, the person may inevitably become a perpetrator again. So, when we use the term "trauma victim," we might actually be referring to both the perpetrator and the victim; they are in one another, true to the teaching of interbeing.

Learn to say sorry to ourselves: "I'm sorry. I have neglected you. I did not get enough sleep. I did not eat healthy food. I had negative thoughts of harming myself, of rejecting myself. For all these, I am very sorry." We need to be able to do this for ourselves, for true healing to be possible. Do not be a hero or a martyr, trying to change others and society, while being oblivious or careless of the fundamental truth that we cannot give what we do not have.

If we cannot confront the demons within and transform our own trauma, how can we change society or the world? I know an American peace activist who is so angry at her country and her government that she refuses to live in the United States. She lives abroad instead, but in this position as an angry peace activist, she is unable to effect change.

3. *It Hurts*

The third part of Beginning Anew is expressing hurts. The body expresses hurts all the time. If we listen, we will recognize that the body is telling us everything that we wish to hear and not wish to hear. For trauma survivors, the mind may consciously or unconsciously suppress the memory of the trauma, so we are not able to fully verbalize or mentally process what we have gone through. Yet, the body itself always speaks truthfully.

As a child, I suffered verbal and physical abuse from my mother. When she was furious, she would beat me or hurl things at me as if I were some despicable creature—a centipede to stomp on. I would stare at her without crying or begging her to stop. Years later I found out from my aunt that after each beating, my mother would quietly rub green oil on my bruises while I was sleeping, muttering, "My poor child, if you were not so stubborn and defiant, I would not have been so enraged and beaten you like this!" My mother did experience remorse, in her own way. I have spent my life learning Beginning Anew to be able to express my hurt to her, and even though she is no longer present physically, the relationship between us has transformed within me, bringing about genuine peace and healing.

4. Resolution

The fourth step of Beginning Anew is finding resolutions. This is about making peace and finding a way out. We all have suffered to a certain extent from various sorts of trauma, whether verbal, physical, sexual, psychological, or ideological. How can we make peace with our trauma and go forward? The way out is in, applying the practice in our daily life so that we can transform our negative habits in ourselves and in our relationships, not repeating the hurts and pains anymore. We can make certain contracts with ourselves like, "I will practice mindfulness while working on the computer, so that I don't ingest toxic items that cause me to get depressed or restless afterward." Or, "When I am angry, I will not say anything, but I will practice walking meditation."

The way out is to have the insight of interbeing, to understand the truth of Thich Nhat Hanh's statement, "Peace in oneself, peace in the world." Peace, self-understanding, self-love, and self-forgiveness enable us to truly reconcile with ourselves and mend the damage that has been caused out of unmindfulness, misunderstanding, misperception, pain, and confusion.

Embracing Instead of Burying Grief: "I Try to Forget My Father"

A short while ago, I met Nhi, a girl of ten years old whose father had killed himself. They'd had a good relationship, but he had been troubled for some time. She saw, in her mind, her father lying dead in their living room. Consequently, she suffered from insomnia. She suffered from chest pains. She was not able to play with her friends, to look her mother in the eye, or to talk to her mother about what she was going through.

"Where do you feel your pain?" I asked her.

"Right here!" she replied, pointing at the middle of her chest. "It feels very heavy here. I cannot sleep at night." Then she went on, "I don't need anybody. I don't like to play with other kids anymore, because I know they won't like me, seeing that I am always sad and keep thinking about my dad. They're scared to talk to me about my dad. Maybe they are afraid that his spirit could still be hanging around me. I don't want to be near my mom either, because one day she will leave me too."

I held her hand tenderly. How many of us, before bringing a child into this world, reflect on our capability to raise this fragile life and think about the legacy we will leave? I thought of her father with compassion. How can a person in trauma take care of his family when he does not even know how to take care of himself? One day, unexpectedly facing an overwhelming situation, he must have fallen into panic and despair, and not knowing what to do, he must have considered suicide as the best solution. He might have thought that death would exempt him from all afflictions, not realizing that death would destroy his physical body but would not erase the unhappiness and suffering caused to his loved ones by his action, speech, and thoughts. This little girl now had to carry the heavy burden her father left behind.

I asked her, "Do you think about your father?"

Nhi replied bleakly, "No. I try to forget him so that I can focus on my studies." This ten-year-old child was already using her studies to bury her pain. This was her coping mechanism!

All of us have done this to ourselves to some degree. When we experience something overwhelming, indescribable, unspeakable to us, we try to suppress it. We try to forget it. The mind can actually compartmentalize it and block it out of its awareness.

However, there is a degree of violence in this action of suppressing our strong emotions. As we have already seen in chapter 1 on mindfulness, the truth is that the undercurrent of deep pain continues to flow after we deny our feelings, like a river that runs underground. The forgetting occurs at the level of the mind consciousness, the mind's surface layer of awareness. Trauma continues to play out in the store consciousness, and it will surge in the body, as chest pain, indigestion, headaches, insomnia; in the feelings, including sadness, fatigue, anxiety, fear, and anger. It will also manifest as mental formations such as nagging, intrusive thoughts and dreams.

In the case of this young child, she was not able to concentrate on her studies or to connect with friends. I advised her, "Please don't try to forget your father. Don't let him die. Keep him alive. He is in you. Every day you can sit with him for five minutes. When you wake up in the morning, just lie there, massage your face, massage your chest, and say, 'Hello Daddy, I know you are there. You are with me still.'"

Then I asked her, "Which parts of you look like your father?"

She replied, "My face looks like my father. My hands look just like my father's hands, and my feet too. I have the legs of my mother and the feet of my father!" Her face brightened when she shared this, as she realized that her father was still alive in her.

I said, "Massage your face and smile to your father. Thank him for the face that he has given you. Hold your own hand and smile to your hands that are the hands of your father. Walk and feel the earth with your feet and say, 'Daddy, I walk for you.'"

In this way, Nhi and I found ways for her to grieve, to remember her father with love, alive and vibrant, supporting the flow of her emotions and her life.

🌸 *Practice: Befriending Our Grief, Keeping Our Beloved Alive*

Read the poem below and breathe with awareness as you read. You can read one line, and then follow your in-breaths and out-breaths for a while before you move on to the next line.

> This breath is for you.
> This smile is for you.
> This peaceful moment is for you.
>
> I breathe for you.
> I smile for you.
> I cultivate this peaceful moment for you.

I am here.

I am here.

I am here.

I am here in this breath.

I am here in this smile.

I am here in this peaceful moment.

I am this breath.

I am this smile.

I am this peaceful moment.

You are life without boundaries.

I am life without boundaries.

Our Loved Ones Live On in Us

If you lose somebody, and you are drowned in sadness, in sorrow, and in forgetfulness, then inadvertently you are making sure that person is as dead as possible. Every time you think about that person, you only think of his or her death. You only think of the person in the past tense. In our practice, we learn to keep our beloved ones alive. I learned to say to my mother, "Mother, I am living stably and beautifully for you. In the thirty-six years of your life, you never really had a chance to sit peacefully. You had to hustle. You had to work so hard to take care of your whole family. Mother, I walk for you. You are alive in me."

Sometimes, our grief is complicated. Our parents may not have always been there for us. They may have been abusive. We may feel a mixture of love and aversion toward them. In meditation, we practice being both kind and truthful, stopping the mind from running away from the present reality or getting hijacked by past memories. We learn to bring the mind back to the here and now, where life is real, and where we have choices in what we do, say, and think. True to the teaching of interbeing, in the present moment there is the past, and there is the future. We don't have to run back to the past to find safety. We don't have to run toward the future either. Dwelling securely in the present moment, we will see clearly what we need to do and not do.

We are the way we are because our fathers and mothers were the way they were. We are not stable because they were not stable. They were not emotionally available for us, and they were not able to handle their own pain and sorrow. That is why now we may still be running away from or drowning in their despair and helplessness. Embracing the wounded child in ourselves, we also acknowledge that our mothers and fathers were children with their own vulnerabilities and traumas. Fortunately, we now have the Five Strengths of self-trust, diligent practice, mindfulness, the transformative power of concentration, and the insight of interbeing. We recognize that with our choices today, we can heal ourselves and we can heal our parents—and all our ancestors—through ourselves.

🌸 Practice: Embracing the Wounded Child in Ourselves and Our Parents

In guided meditation, one line is recited for the in-breath and another line is recited for the out-breath. If the line is long, then you can silently recite it as you are breathing in and out mindfully. Each exercise is shortened by key words, which may help you focus your mind so that you can continue to follow your breathing as you practice looking deeply. Each guided phrase may last two minutes or however long it may take you to feel in touch and at ease with that part of the meditation. I also shared this practice of embracing the child within ourselves and within our parents in *Mindfulness as Medicine*.

Remember that meditation is like a bird with two wings—one is stopping and the other deep looking. In sitting meditation, whether it is silent or guided, we always start with stopping. We stop the mind from ceaseless thinking and aimless wandering by bringing the mind back, first to the breathing, and then to the body. Once the mind is anchored stably in the breath and body in the here and now, we can proceed to the second wing of meditation with a specific topic for contemplation.

1. First, practice stopping by being aware of the breath.
   - Breathing in, I am aware that I am breathing in.
     Breathing out, I am aware that I am breathing out.
     In-breath
     Out-breath
   - Breathing in, I follow my in-breath from the beginning to
        the end.
     Breathing out, I follow my out-breath from the beginning to
        the end.
     Following in-breath
     Following out-breath

2. Practice stopping by being aware of the body.
   - Breathing in, I am aware that I have a body.
     Breathing out, I smile to my body.
     Aware of body
     Smiling to body

- Breathing in, I am aware of the pain and tension in certain parts of my body.

  Breathing out, I smile and release tension from each part of my body.

  Aware of tension and pain

  Releasing

3. Practice looking deeply.

   - Breathing in, I see myself as a child.

     Breathing out, I smile to the child that is still alive in me.

     Seeing myself as a child

     Smiling

     Hello, my inner child

   - Breathing in, I see the child in me as fragile, vulnerable, experiencing certain hurts and pains.

     Breathing out, I smile and embrace my inner child with my stable posture and mindful breathing.

     Seeing the child fragile and vulnerable

     Embracing

     I am here for you.

   - Breathing in, I recognize that my childhood trauma continues to manifest in my daily life through my thoughts, speech, and bodily actions.

     Breathing out, I smile and embrace my inner child with my stable posture and mindful breathing.

     Recognizing my inner child alive in me

     Embracing

     I hear you! I see you!

- Breathing in, I'm aware that I am older now, with many positive conditions for practicing, healing, and transforming my inner child.

  Breathing out, I feel hope and confidence in myself.

  Aware of positive conditions

  Feeling hopeful and confident

  Thank you!

- Breathing in, joy is in each mindful in-breath.

  Breathing out, healing is in each mindful out-breath

  Joy

  Healing

  Breathe. I am alive!

In the same sitting meditation session, after you have looked deeply into yourself as a child, you can move on to look deeply into your father as a child, and then into your mother as a child. Many teenagers have reported that this guided meditation helps them to see their parents, for the first time, as children, fragile, vulnerable, and having suffering of their own. You may not be able to contemplate yourself or your parents as children in the first session. You may cry or freeze because so much pain arises. In this case, stay with the breathing and maintain a stable posture. You can also stop this meditation and go back to it another time when you feel more ready. As you practice this guided meditation a few times, you will experience more empathy and understanding for your parents.

You may also choose to look deeply into the child in yourself, in your father, and in your mother in separate sitting sessions. If this is the case, the steps are still the same. Go through step 1-2 above, bringing the mind back to the breath and the body, then move to step 3, looking deeply into the inner child in our father or mother.

- Breathing in, I see my father/mother as a child.

  Breathing out, I smile to the child that is still alive in my father/mother.

  Seeing my father/mother as a child, smiling

- Breathing in, I see the child in my father/mother as fragile and as having certain struggles and difficulties.

  Breathing out, I smile and embrace the child in my father/mother with my stable posture and mindful breathing.

  Seeing the child fragile, vulnerable, and struggling

  Embracing

- Breathing in, I recognize that the child's fragility, vulnerability, struggles, and difficulties continue to manifest in my daily life through my thoughts, speech, and bodily actions.

  Breathing out, I smile and embrace the child in my father/mother in me with my stable posture and mindful breathing.

  Recognizing the child of father/mother alive in me

  Embracing

- Breathing in, I am aware that I am an adult now, with many positive conditions to practice, heal, and transform my father's/mother's inner child in me.

  Breathing out, I feel hope and confidence in myself.

  Aware of positive conditions

  Feeling hopeful and confident

- Breathing in, each mindful in-breath is joy and healing.

  Breathing out, each mindful out-breath is joy and healing.

  Joy in each breath

  Healing in each breath

🌸 Practice: *Wielding a Mantra*

A mantra is a sacred utterance believed to have religious, magical, or spiritual powers in Eastern religions. Thich Nhat Hanh taught us many wonderful mantras in English, and over the years, I have also concocted some on my own. I offer a few below. They sound so simple, but they truly work! Of course, you may not be able to wield the magic at first, so it takes patience and practice. Follow your breath a few times before you say a mantra with as much sincerity and clarity as you can. They can have a profound positive effect on your body and mind as soon as you pronounce them. As you practice these mantras diligently, they replace your habitual negative thoughts and feelings. For example, instead of thinking, "I'm bored," "It's horrible!" and suffering through a painful situation, saying the mantra, "I am here for you," or "Smile, my dear" and aligning yourself with it will dispel your negative thoughts and empower you to face your circumstances with a more balanced mind.

Here are some simple mantras to say to yourself, to help you overcome difficulties. In time, you can formulate some more mantras that you can tailor to your personality and situation.

When you are anxious or stressed
Breathe. It'll be okay.
Smile, my dear.
I am here for you.
I am okay.
I love you so!

When you recognize you need to take care of yourself
Help me to take better care of you.
Thank you for trying. Thank you for doing your best.
I am sorry.
Thank you.

When you are aware your thoughts are negative or "stuck"

Are you sure?
If you are sure, check again.
This, too, will pass.

When you are rushing

This is a happy moment!
Oh, my happiness!
I am beautiful!
I am enough!
I am so blessed!
I am whole!

PART 3

THE *five* MINDFULNESS TRAININGS AS A *source* OF STRENGTH

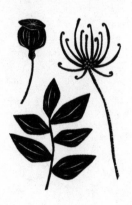

CHAPTER 8

Reverence for Life

To gain the strength to reclaim our power to heal, it is vital to have proper guidance for living a happy life. But many of us don't actually know what that looks like. Today we tend to look to science for answers rather than religion, to clinicians rather than priests. Systems such as Buddhism are a source of tried and tested wisdom that combine the ethical with the scientific. When we talk about the five precepts of traditional Buddhism in Plum Village, we call them the "Five Mindfulness Trainings," because they are concrete expressions, manifestations of mindfulness that we can apply—and, most important, *train in and practice* in our daily life. These five areas of training have been refined by generations of practitioners as the practical basis of a happy, meaningful, and liberatory life.

Rather than a moral code that we must believe and stick to blindly, we practice the trainings and observe the benefits. It is like training in a martial art like aikido; there's no use just looking at the list of principles. We commit ourselves to the training with diligence to increase our strength and resiliency in order to heal past traumas, to prevent creating further traumas, and to live our life with renewed intention each day. These trainings can be approached as a path, a way of life, as well as a source of spiritual sustenance. They serve as the North Star, guiding our thoughts, speech, and bodily actions in accordance with our wish for peace, healing, and transformation. They are a mirror in which we can see our states of mind, and discern whether our actions stem from conscious choice or from habit energy.

For survivors of trauma, they can serve as a moral compass to help us through the healing process.

The Five Mindfulness Trainings

1. Reverence for Life
2. True Happiness
3. True Love
4. Loving Speech and Deep Listening
5. Nourishment and Healing

People often think the first mindfulness training of Reverence for Life correlates to the biblical commandment "Thou shalt not kill" and is about being vegetarian, avoiding crushing insects when we walk, and so on—but in truth it's about holding our own life with love and respect first and foremost. By not neglecting, abusing, or hurting ourself, we learn to cherish ourself, and to be grateful for our body—for our "one wild and precious life," as Mary Oliver would say. We do our best to take care of ourselves.

Reverence for Life also means being aware of the awesome power, constructive as well as destructive, of our thoughts, speech, and bodily actions and wield this power in the direction always nurturing life—our own life and the lives of other people and species. So we do not dismiss our mental activities, saying "A thought is just a thought," because we know that a thought can influence our speech and bodily actions now and for generations to come. We don't rehearse negative thinking; we don't water those seeds of self-destructiveness, discrimination, and hatred. Therefore, we become more responsible for our views and mindsets.

The second mindfulness training is True Happiness. In the context of trauma, when we suffer we only see conditions of suffering, of despair. We replay our past suffering. When we realize that True Happiness is right here and right now and not in external conditions, we can let go of the past and be grateful for what we do have. We embrace our past suffering, but we don't rehearse it. We fully grieve what has been lost to us, but we live in the present. Actively, in each moment, we can choose how to think, how to speak, how to behave—how to take care of the situation as it comes in the form of the present moment. We train ourselves to respond to current conditions appropriately instead of reacting to them like we are a victim in the past.

True happiness also means that we know we have enough. We learn to live a simple lifestyle, not investing anxious energy and effort in an effort to ensure happiness in the future.

Knowing we don't have to be in control of everything, and having a strong sense of trust in ourselves, we let go of our hypervigilance and fear. So many of us delay our happiness with thoughts like, *I'll be safe and happy if I'm successful, if I get into the right university, if I have a great partner,* and we keep running away from all the conditions of happiness available here right now. So we learn to recognize what we already have and cherish it. This gives us energy and hope, to do what we need to do in the world.

The third mindfulness training, True Love, is correlated to the traditional Buddhist precept about refraining from sexual misconduct, so, it is directly concerned with sexual trauma. The Buddha taught that sexual energy, breath energy, and spiritual energy interrelate, one transforming into and affecting the other. It is a different view of human sexuality than what is promoted in our culture's norms. In my book *Mindfulness as Medicine*, I put forward interbeing, healing, friendship, joy, respect, and trust as the six basic elements of True Love—if these six elements are not present in your relationship with another person, then it is not a truly loving relationship.

Many of us may be confused by sexual energy—not just those who have experienced childhood sexual trauma. Because our culture has become so hypersexualized, many people don't know how to relate to each other in a wholesome way. In a sense, we have all been exposed to sexual trauma, through our mass media; scenes of sexual violence are common in "entertainment."

We aren't conscious that our breath and our spiritual and sexual energies are related, and we have no idea how to channel our sexual energy into spiritual energy that nourishes us and nurtures our friendships. If we are steady meditators, with mindfulness, concentration, and insight, we have the capacity to channel our sexual energy into breath energy and spiritual energy for our own protection and freedom.

The fourth mindfulness training is Loving Speech and Deep Listening. Again, we include ourselves as recipients of the benefits of this training. When we say to ourselves, *It's okay, I'm here for you*, we are practicing loving speech. When we do sitting meditation, we are practicing deep listening to ourselves, to our inner child. Whenever we make mistakes, we don't put ourselves down. We gently ask ourselves, *Please help me to understand why I react in such a way. What does it mean?* These are all practices of Loving Speech and Deep Listening. So, every mindfulness training is a loving practice. When we walk mindfully, we listen to our steps, and we realize when we're angry, we're pounding on the earth. But when we're at peace, our steps are gentle, quiet. When we are angry, and we do walking meditation, then we're not pounding on the ground; we're not hurting our body, but we're also not rehearsing the suffering. So loving speech and deep listening take place throughout the day, bringing about many moments of enlightenment, and the transformation of habits and pains. Whatever arises, we say, "It's okay, we'll take care of one thing at a time."

The fifth training is on Nourishment and Healing, also known as mindful consumption. This is mindful consumption of our own thoughts, feelings, perspectives; mindful consumption of our speech toward ourselves, positive or negative, beneficial or harmful. We need to know when to change the song of our self-talk when it gets negative. If we say to ourselves, *You are stupid,* we can then say, *I'm sorry,* and begin anew right away with ourselves. We say thank you to ourselves, and thank you to others. Mindful consumption is starting fresh with ourselves, daily, moment to moment. When we have a bad day, when we suffer, we tend to go to movies, to games, to escape. That's okay for a temporary fix, but ultimately we need to be aware of our patterns. Usually we develop coping mechanisms in our childhood; we find a way to cope, or to escape the situation. Then it becomes a perpetual pattern, a personality, a destiny.

Many of our coping mechanisms since childhood or our teenage years may be negative. Our practice is to be there for what is, not to escape. We need to teach our children ways of being with what is. To hold and embrace. To soothe, then to look into the situation and find a way out—as soon as possible. Not to let ourselves escape, year after year. That's mindful consumption: to learn to transform our negative coping mechanisms into positive, constructive approaches; to breathe with awareness when stressed; when suffering arises, to walk with it and look into it deeply, so that we may truly engage with life.

The First Mindfulness Training: Reverence For Life

Aware of the suffering caused by the destruction of life,
I am committed to cultivating the insight of interbeing

and compassion and learning ways to protect the lives of people, animals, plants, and minerals. I am determined not to kill, not to let others kill, and not to support any act of killing in the world, in my thinking, or in my way of life. Seeing that harmful actions arise from anger, fear, greed, and intolerance, which in turn come from dualistic and discriminative thinking, I will cultivate openness, non-discrimination, and non-attachment to views in order to transform violence, fanaticism, and dogmatism in myself and in the world.

The basis of mindfulness is reverence for life. The sexual abuse I suffered as a child affected all facets all my life, without my conscious awareness. One way it manifested was in powerful, overwhelming, relentless thoughts of harming myself and ending my life, what psychologists call "suicidal ideation."

From the age of nine into adulthood, I frequently fantasized about suicide. This may be difficult for people who have not experienced severe trauma to understand, but it is common for trauma survivors to battle with thoughts of ending our lives. We may believe it an ideal solution to mental suffering, a magical way out of the abyss of our pain and confusion. Perversely, I believed death was my only real friend and confidant since childhood, listening to me and comforting me, "I know. I know. You can count on me. I am always here for you!"

In many countries, suicide is a leading cause of death among young people. We resort to self-harm and suicide when we do not know how to handle our strong emotions and the suffering in our life. Developing the Five Strengths, which empower us, we learn to turn away before we reach such despair, and not feed despairing thoughts that would lead us to that point.

An Autobiography of Suicidal Thinking

As a nine-year-old girl in Saigon, coinciding with the time of the abuse by my uncle, I would bite my nails so much that when I washed my hands it felt like electric shocks, they were so sore. The skin underneath my nails would bleed and be painful. Later, I started to pull my hair and even caused a bald spot, which caused me much embarrassment when a boy in my class yelled out in front of everyone, "Look at her! She is bald!" I would obsessively try to cover the bald spot with the help of hairpins. Many years later in medical school, I learned the medical terminology for my behavior, *trichotillomania*—compulsive hair-pulling to neutralize an anxious feeling from stress and trauma—and I realized that I was not alone in this behavior.

Suicidal thoughts became more frequent in my early teenage years. Saigon is a city of many rivers and bridges, and every time I passed one I would visualize myself jumping into the water. The impulse was strong and alluring.

I attempted suicide at age fifteen. It started out with something ridiculously small. Grandma had bought me a pair of shoes, and I wanted to wear them since my old pair was so worn out. Out of nowhere, my uncle sneered at me, "She just wants to look attractive to the boys." His statement suddenly triggered something violent in me. Consciously, I did not understand it, but subconsciously something was triggered.

I ran upstairs and found my mother's bottle of pills. She had disappeared three years previously and left a bottle of painkillers. I swallowed all the pills—about thirty of them. Then I came downstairs and sat facing my uncle, defying him.

"Okay, now I will die, and I hope that satisfies you," I said.

Alarmed by my statement, my grandmother asked, "What do you mean by that?"

I directed my answer to my uncle. "You ruined my life."

That was the very first time I ever said anything to my uncle about his sexual abuse, not fully aware of the implications of my own statement. Again, Grandma looked at me, very concerned, and repeated, "What do you mean by that?" My uncle stayed silent and he left the room.

I sat there waiting to die.

Most likely because the medication was outdated, nothing happened to me, not even a minor stomachache or nausea! It was anticlimactic and disappointing! Life went on as usual. Nevertheless, the powerful thoughts and feelings remained deeply etched in me just the same: *I attempted suicide at age of fifteen. I could have died then.* Looking back, I appreciate Grandma's concern and willingness to ask questions, and I wonder what might have shifted in the course of my life if I could have told her about the abuse then. But I did not speak about it further.

The following year, when I turned sixteen, I began to have the strong belief that I would die at twenty-six. This belief persisted into my college years and into medical school, when I started to write a living will every year. I would have my best friend sign it. In my living will, she would get all my journals, and the few thousand dollars I had in the bank would go to my brother, Sonny. I was always more prepared to die than to live. I did not realize that not all my peers were doing the same thing.

Suicidal thoughts had become habitual as I grew older—they were my norm. Every time I had difficulties—particularly in relationships, or when I was depressed or under severe stress—death served as my default solution; my mind would jump quickly to the thought *I can just die, and all this will stop.* I never attempted suicide again, but those thoughts were always there.

In college, I put up a full-length poster on my dorm door for Halloween, and then left it up for the whole year. On it, I had cut out an image of a man holding up a mask, with a black background and red cursive arching over him: "I waver between the living and the dead." Talk about watering unwholesome seeds and suicidal thoughts in myself! Imagine, seeing those words daily on my door for a year! Unbeknownst to me, my store consciousness was informing me that I was literally wavering between the living and the dead for most of my life.

Even if perpetrators of sexual violence do not take the life of their victims, they may have effectively killed or stifled the desire to live in them. Many survivors "waver between the living and the dead" throughout their lives, until they have a chance to heal themselves. The abusers have also killed their own compassion and their clear conscience, as they fall victim to the darkness lurking in their mind.

Frequently, in my dreams, I would be chased and pushed down, and would wake up screaming. In college, I had a dream in which I saw myself walking by a group of men, and one reached out to grab me. I hit him back so hard that I woke up instantly with a jolt. I had hit the edge of the table next to my bed. The tabletop was marble, so I got an immediate hematoma. Another time, I woke up next to my boyfriend and saw that he was in tears. He told me that he was trying to hold me while I was sleeping, but I repeatedly pushed him away and kicked him! I had no awareness of my actions, which were so hurtful to him.

When I was about to turn twenty-six, I was in my second year of medical school in San Francisco, seemingly with everything to live for. I said to my best friend, Jennifer, that I would probably die that year. I had been ready for it all these years. She took me very seriously. A spiritual person in her own way, Jennifer told me, "Can you ask the higher power, God and Buddha, to extend your life, because you have much to give in this life? You have a lot to do still. Please ask for more time."

We went to a quiet place on Potrero Hill and sat side by side and looked out over the city. Then I asked for more time in this world. "Dear Buddha, if you can give me more time to live, I will do my best to live beautifully and to help other people." As I was training to be a doctor at the time, my medical career was my sense of purpose.

For my twenty-sixth birthday, I hosted a gathering of thirty good friends from college and medical school. They shared how I had affected their lives, in glowing terms—as if they were giving me eulogies. This happened again the night before I graduated from medical school, when many good friends came and shared beautiful memories of the positive influences I had on their lives. These outpourings of love and affection fed my soul and gave me a reason to continue on my path. So I lived on, finished medical school, and went on to my residency.

Not until much later in my life did I ask myself, *Why did I think I would die at twenty-six? Was it a conscious or unconscious wish?* Gradually an insight came to me. Life had been interminable and unbearable for the wounded child in me, who saw no hope as she was growing into a teenager. So her mind resolved the dilemma by giving her a deadline of age twenty-six, literally a *dead*-line, which then made life seem more bearable, because there would be an end to it all. The thought there would be an end to this life of suffering was like medicine, providing deep comfort.

All my life I had told myself, after all the suffering I had had to endure in my childhood, if I could just become successful and find somebody who loved me and whom I loved back, then it would make up for all the pain, loneliness, and despair that I experienced as a child. The deep scars of being born in a country at war, abused by my uncle, having a mother who was murdered, losing my grandma, and growing up as an orphan in America could somehow be healed through romantic love. Yet here I was, a doctor with a loving partner, still drowning in my own suffering and despair!

When my beloved John died suddenly, I touched the depths of despair again. For days I tried to make sense of my suffering by driving on the freeway. I would wake up early in the morning, get in the car, and race on the highway along the ocean and the cliffs near San Francisco, my mind filled with the obsessive impulse to swerve the car into one of those cliffs. It would just take just a second to swerve the car, and I would be free from the torture of being alive. I wouldn't have to face suffering or feel anything anymore. Losing a partner, someone I loved and cherished, was agonizing, but I was also devastated from losing all my dreams.

When somebody you love dies suddenly, the pain is harrowing. Of course, this is because of the attachment you have for the person, but their death also causes you to face your own life. *How have I lived my life? If I were to die in the middle of the day now, can I say that I have lived fully? What would I leave behind?*

John was somebody who had lived a joyful, spiritual, and meaningful life. When I was with him, I wasn't an inwardly focused person. I was so wrapped up in my work, my unresolved trauma and stress, my own sadness and despair, that many times I actually pushed him away. The day that he died, we were supposed to meet with each other to celebrate my birthday, but I had told him I couldn't make it, because I was too busy with work in the hospital. It was true that I was on call, but it was also true that I was intentionally avoiding him. His sudden death, as a result, inundated me not only with grief but also with unbearable guilt and regret.

I had met Thich Nhat Hanh and the mindfulness practice a few weeks before my partner's death. This encounter gave me the hope of finding inner peace, despite the pain of my past. With the insight of interbeing, I later realized: If I were to die in despair, would my suffering really go away? Sure, the body would be destroyed. But the suffering itself would live on—in my brother, in his children, in my relatives, in those who knew me, in the consciousness of the world and of the cosmos.

Saved by One Breath

Even after I had become a nun and was practicing mindfulness daily, I noticed a familiar pattern to my thinking. Early in my monastic practice, I had learned to become more aware of the habitual, automatic nature of my death wish, and how to breathe with it and release it, but recurring thoughts of my partner's death intensified my depression and the desire to end my life.

The turning point was an incident I shared in my memoir, *Healing*, when I had a breakdown. I was walking in the forest near Plum Village's Lower Hamlet. The burden of suffering was so heavy in my chest that I could not breathe, and the act of screaming seemed to release that suffocating energy. I began crying and screaming at the top of my lungs. At one point, a flash of knowing came to me, that I was about to step over the boundary between sanity and insanity. I saw it so quickly and clearly in that moment.

Immediately, I took in the deepest breath of my life, gulping for air with my mouth wide open. I collapsed among the quiet trees. On my hands and knees, I started to pray, "Please, please, help me never to suffer again, never to go to this dark place again." I prayed for my life, to come back from the dead.

One moment before, I had been completely swept away by my feelings and emotions. But that deep breath brought me back to my body, to that moment, and to my deepest desire to transform my suffering and not to be a victim anymore.

Soon after that, two sisters appeared. A group of nuns and lay friends had been walking along the road by the wood and heard frightening inhuman-sounding cries. They could not figure out what kind of animal could produce such excruciating sounds of pain and went to investigate. Two brave sisters actually came right up to the source of the sound and found me lying on the ground in a state of exhaustion. One on each side, they led me back to my room. Sister Tín Nghiêm, a Korean sister, sat with me for a long time. She sang quietly Thay's poem "For Warmth" to me:

> I hold my face in my two hands.
> No, I am not crying.
> I hold my face in my two hands
> to keep the loneliness warm—
> two hands protecting,
> two hands nourishing,
> two hands preventing
> my soul from leaving me
> in anger.

While my Sister continued to sing the song over and over again, I lay there curled up in a ball, slowly returning to normalcy. That was the most dramatic incident I had, right at the threshold of insanity. I have never gone there again.

I wrote the following poem in gratitude in the memory of John.

HOLDING MY FACE

I cried in bed last night
Things I shared of my heart now
Lay open in the eyes of others
I dared not look at them.

My quiet sister held me
From her bed, singing:
"I hold my face in my two hands,
To catch what might fall from within
Deeper than crying
I am not crying...."

I hold my face in my two hands
So that when I look up
I see my true face
And the face of my beloved.

Healing Our Negative Thoughts

Ten years after ordination, I contracted Lyme disease. It had a debilitating effect on my health and energy. I recognized the return of certain repetitive thoughts: *Everything is out of control. Life is not worth living. I am not worth keeping alive.* Even if we do not actually take our life, such messages themselves are devastating for the psyche, as I explained in chapter 1, as well as for the immune system and for the entire body, making us more vulnerable to illnesses. This kind of self-destructive thinking drains our life energy and our capacity for healing.

Having developed a greater capacity for mindfulness, I began to see much earlier how the emotions and the suicidal thoughts were building up their momentum. I would breathe, relax, and smile to them as if to old friends, gently humoring myself, saying, *I am dying anyway, I don't have to wish for death.*

WAITING TO DIE

Sometimes I sit waiting to die,
While marveling at the evening light glowing over treetops,
Watching an ant scurrying to and fro,
And listening to young birds' calls, near and far.

I know that life is like a waterfall.
My body grows older and weaker every moment.
I know that my own mind creates afflictions,
Grasping for rain bubbles this entire human life.

Still, sometimes I sit waiting to die.
Death sings each in-breath and out-breath!

Let the thoughts of love and rejection exhibit themselves.
Let the dust fly. Just watch it fly.
Keep on breathing, smiling, and waiting to die.
Be present to understand this "I" more.
Ah, the moment without waiting!
There is no coming, no going.

The body is always living and dying as part of a natural process. Old cells die and new cells are regenerated, most visibly seen in skin and hair cells. I do not have to wish for death. It will happen naturally. *May I learn to live meaningfully and beautifully. May I learn to die beautifully, each day.* Thus, I have learned to transform my suicidal thoughts.

In living our life beautifully, we touch death beautifully. Otherwise, life and death are only notions—we may grasp one and reject the other, without ever knowing what they are truly about. To heal these suicidal thoughts means to gain control, confidence, and love for oneself and for one's life. We learn to release the tension in the body, in the feelings and the thoughts, caring for ourselves, instead of deserting ourselves or being swept under by a strong current of despair. Slowly we regain faith in ourselves and experience more optimism in life. To be able to see a purple flower blooming through the cracks on the sidewalk. The sunrise. The faces of our loved ones. To know that they are there. To acknowledge, "I am still alive, and you are still there." To greet our body, "Hello, my eyes, I know you are there, and I am thankful. Hello, my heart, I am grateful that you are still beating. Hello, my liver, I am sorry for having been unkind to you. Thank you for helping me to eat healthier, to not consume drugs and alcohol anymore."

It is a simple relief to receive comfort in Mother Earth while sitting on a rock, while lying under a tree's canopy, while walking with relaxed steps, knowing that Mother Earth is always there to embrace us, in life and in death. Peace of mind is there when we realize there is no need to grasp for release.

We Are All Connected

I have learned to heal the wounded child in me, whose only way to escape from the pain of life was to fantasize about death. Suicide serves as a romantic escape in theory, but in truth it only perpetuates more pain and drama. Without a path out of suffering, our friends and loved ones will have to carry the unresolved pain of our death and their feelings of loss and despair for the rest of their lives. That is the wheel of samsara, the cycle of death and rebirth, of suffering and pain being transmitted from one person to another, one generation to the next, with no exit.

The insight of interbeing can help heal our individualism, loneliness, and despair. I see many young people nowadays who are depressed, suffering from anxiety and suicidal ideation when their problems seem unbearable or insurmountable, just like I once did. When we have an incorrect view about the self, we may think, *This is my body. I can do whatever I want with it.* Even sincere Buddhist practitioners who value animal and plant life can be neglectful and abusive of their own bodies. We may use this very body to punish someone else or to punish ourselves.

When we gain the insight of interbeing, we see that this body is not our body. This body is a transmission from our father, mother, grandparents, and generations of ancestors. They have given us this body and entrusted us with it. We are continuing *them*. Reverence for Life allows us to have gratitude for our ancestors' gift to us, this unique existence.

CHAPTER 9

True Happiness

In Clarity Hamlet in Deer Park Monastery, there used to live an elderly nun in her seventies, whom I called Sư Má ("Teacher Mother") because she treated me like her own daughter. She would often save some goodies for me or give me a red envelope on the first day of the Lunar New Year. One time she called me into her room and gave me a pack of underwear, making a big fuss of me and saying, "My daughter sent them to me, but I have enough already. Please keep them for your own use." I was so moved by her thoughtfulness, I thanked her and hugged her. Later, a thought dawned on me, *Oh dear, I am wearing old ladies' underwear! What has happened to me?* I had once been quite selective about the clothes I wore. It was bittersweet. Still, I happily wore them for many years.

A happy life starts with simplicity in material things. How does this relate to trauma? Happiness, real happiness, is healing. The sense of contentment we gain from cultivating contentment in a world of duality and opposites is supportive of our healing. Having a less materially focused life helps us have more mental space for ourselves. Instead of craving new things, we develop more equanimity and peace of mind.

The Second Mindfulness Training: True Happiness

Aware of the suffering caused by exploitation, social injustice, stealing, and oppression, I am committed to practicing generosity in my thinking, speaking, and acting. I am determined not to steal and not to possess anything that should belong to others; and I will share my time, energy, and material resources with those who are in need. I will practice looking deeply to see that the happiness and suffering of others are not separate from my own happiness and suffering; that true happiness is not possible without understanding and compassion; and that running after wealth, fame, power, and sensual pleasures can bring much suffering and despair. I am aware that happiness depends on my mental attitude and not on external conditions, and that I can live happily in the present moment simply by remembering that I already have more than enough conditions to be happy. I am committed to practicing Right Livelihood so that I can help reduce the suffering of living beings on Earth and stop contributing to climate change.

A Monastic Approach to Material and Emotional Decluttering

I recommend cleaning the house often and giving away things that you have not used in a year; somebody else can make better use of it. Clear your garage of unused items. As nuns and monks, we just have the space under our bed, which we call a "bed box" to store our things, and still we can accumulate a lot. Every year, at the start of our three-month Rains Retreats, we review our possessions and pass on items we no longer need, and we find we always have more than enough.

I go through my belongings all the time, at least once every two months. When I see somebody with a lot of stuff, it inspires me to come back to my room and clear more away. When you simplify your life outwardly, you are actually learning to simplify your life inwardly. If you want to go buy a new set of clothes or something, ask yourself: *Do I really need it? Sure, I want it, but do I really need it?* Try waiting, and not getting it right away. Learn to look at that desire, hold it, and breathe with it, because in this modern time, we—especially Americans—feel so entitled to everything. The pattern goes: *I want it, so I get it. I have money. I can find it on Google or on Amazon. I buy it online, and it comes the next day.*

This sense of entitlement feeds our ego and all of the pairs of opposites:

I versus you.

New versus old.

Good versus bad.

There is the *me*, there is the *mine*, and I want to satisfy the "me" and make it feel good. When we let go of duality, we access a different kind of feeling good—the goodness of wholeness.

Train to hold off this sense of entitlement and grasping. If you want something, hold the thought of acquiring it and breathe with it three times. Hold it off for a day, a week, a month, or a year. Sometimes in the very next moment, you may not desire it anymore.

As a nun, I have very few clothes. I have one brown robe that I have been wearing the last seventeen years. My auntie had it made and brought it to Plum Village for me in 2003. I have worn this robe every single morning when I go to sitting meditation. I have worn it to most of the Dharma talks that I have offered. There is also a pair of pants that goes with the robe as a set. The pants became so faded and discolored that I asked a sister to sew them inside-out for me. A few days later, another sister asked me, "Where did you get that new pair of pants? They look so dark." I replied, "Actually, these are my old pants, and they've just been sewn inside out." Certainly, I can have another set made, but I keep this robe because it has been with me for seventeen years now. It is my daily practice robe, a witness to a simple life, so that I may invest my energy in the practice, which has yielded the fruit of true peace and long-lasting happiness. My beautiful worldly clothing, however exquisitely tailored and expensive, had only brought me temporary excitement and satisfaction.

We can take the same view with our body. Our body teaches us so much. We can learn to treasure it, however young or old, beautiful or ugly, smooth or wrinkled, healthy or damaged it may be. It is ours, my dear. *And* it is not ours, belonging to our long line of ancestors. Take good care of it. Listen to it, treasure it, send love to it. It will not always be here. Our body changes every moment. And yet—another paradox—there is no coming, no going. Our body is a manifestation of so many conditions, and even as we age and die, we continue in so many ways, forever.

The capacity to cherish what we have and yet not to grasp it brings great happiness. Gratitude generates happiness. It's like going on a hike on a magnificent natural reserve. Our six sense organs can fully enjoy the spaciousness and the beautiful sights and sounds of nature. We feel happy because we are present and free to enjoy all that is there, not because it belongs to us. This is the flavor of True Happiness.

Hoarding Is a Disorder

There are those of us survivors who hoard material things. We keep everything, every memento, every single plastic bag, every box or newspaper, or whatever fits our fancy. Hoarding can become hazardous.

People cannot cook because things are all over their kitchen. There have been instances when people have burned to death inside their homes because they could not find a way out, and the firefighters couldn't find a way in to save them; or when stacks of objects have collapsed on top of a person and they were unable to free themselves. Yet when family members tell a hoarder they have a problem, they do not see it or believe it. They think it is completely normal.

That is hoarding material things. Everybody else can see it, except the hoarders themselves. Have you heard of mental hoarders? Indeed, many of us hoard thoughts about the past and about the future: feelings of sorrow, anger, fear, hatred, jealousy, and regrets; experiences that were pleasant or unpleasant. Who can see those thoughts, feelings, and views? We do not even see them ourselves! Have you ever found yourself recounting the same story or memory to someone who has already heard this story?

Attached and addicted to them, we do not want to let go of even one thought. They are so dear to us that we subconsciously protect our thoughts and feelings from those who try to help us, with the attitude, "Don't you dare to touch my memories and my treasured suffering!" We become exceedingly sensitive and fragile. Strange and even offensive as this may sound, this attachment to our feelings, thoughts, and views is a reality for many of us. We must be able to observe this mental hoarding in our own mind and connect it to our suffering, so as to let go of our stuck views to make room for new thoughts and feelings and a new vitality to take root. Otherwise, our tendency to rehearse suffering may continue to control us and drive our thoughts, speech, and bodily actions. When we are breathing in fresh air, relaxing our body and our thoughts, we may find ourselves smiling with the pairs of opposites that arise constantly throughout the day and throughout our life.

Rebel with a Cause

On one occasion, Thich Nhat Hanh asked me, "My child, are we rebels?" I smiled and replied, "Yes, dear Thay. We are rebels ... with a cause." This was a reference to the movie *Rebel Without a Cause,* starring James Dean. For twenty years now, I have learned to turn inward and be a rebel against my own attachment, restlessness, confusion, and pain, not allowing myself to succumb to them. Keenly aware and grateful that Thay had made deliberate and difficult choices in his life so that many of us might be his spiritual children and benefit from a life of peace and freedom, I have also made the vow to transform my attachment and aversion, to make real the Dharma name Thay gave me on the day of my ordination: Dang Nghiem—nondiscrimination, equanimity—as a path to my true peace and freedom. I have no other wish except to live this life of practice and service until my last breath, and to smile until my last out-breath. Thanks to Thay's love, I may live my life fully and with no regret.

Awareness of our thoughts and feelings gradually enables us to not be pushed or pulled by desire or aversion or other pairs of opposites. There is a great happiness that I never knew existed. I used to believe that if I did not have an object of desire—something to achieve or someone to pursue—then life would be so boring and lonesome. I had pursued both romance and success, and yet I was still quite lonesome, restless, and in despair. To be able to simply sit with oneself, breathe with oneself, be with what is arising within and without, and not being pushed or pulled by it—even if you just touch one moment of this, you will see that it is like a superpower, conferring great happiness and freedom! Then you practice cultivating more of these moments, removing the sense of separateness bit by bit so that you can simply be. Eventually, the duality of what we call right view versus wrong view will not have to be there either.

This is a life work *and* a moment-to-moment practice. It is wonderful to have a spiritual family to take refuge in and to practice with. The mindfulness trainings are concrete practices that help us cultivate peace and true happiness within. Then, if something were to happen and you were to die in the middle of the day, you would not have to regret anything. You would not have to be afraid, because you would know that you have done your best to live as beautifully and to die as beautifully as you can.

Happiness Here and Now

My niece, Sunee, recently asked my best friend's son, a French teenager, "Would you rather read a book or be on a beautiful tropical island?" He responded, "Read a book." She asked, "Would you rather read a book at home or on a beautiful tropical island?" He responded, "I'd rather read a book at home."

"I am comfortable at home," he added.

Many people nowadays do not experience the joy or pleasure of being outdoors in nature. They find exhilaration in the virtual world of books, games, and movies. While being contented to stay home with a book is a wonderful thing, we shouldn't neglect our need for contact with nature. The practice of walking meditation reacquaints us to the sensation of our feet touching the ground, the wind blowing our hair, the sunlight warming our skin. A preoccupied mind does not perceive or appreciate a tenacious little dandelion growing out of the crack on the sidewalk. Yet, when that mind is present and calm, such a dandelion is a sight of awe and inspiration! Happiness is there, right in that moment!

In my daily life, I train myself to do walking meditation wherever I go. A sign that I am mindful is that I am aware of my breath and my steps. Another sign of mindfulness is that I can see and appreciate something interesting or beautiful on the way. If we truly want to be happy, we need to train ourselves to recognize all the beautiful, simple things around us. Otherwise, happiness becomes the carrot hung on the nose of the donkey for it to chase after. It is always something ahead of us, tempting but continually evading us and unattainable.

When we suffer from trauma, we tend to focus only on conditions of suffering and despair, replaying and rehearsing past suffering. The mind is the painter of our world; if the painter only uses dark colors, then all paintings will look dismal and bleak. True happiness is vibrant, right here and right now, within us and all around us. We allow ourselves to acknowledge and be grateful for what we still have, not what has been lost to us. Actively in each moment, with our Five Strengths of trust, energy, mindfulness, concentration, and insight, we can choose how to think, how to speak, how to behave—how to take care of the situation as it manifests in the present moment; how to respond to it proactively and appropriately instead of reacting to it as if we were a victim in the past.

True happiness also means that we know we have enough. We learn to live a simple lifestyle, not trying so hard to accumulate material things, not investing so much of our energy and effort in the future, misled by the false belief that we will be happy when we become successful. Recognizing what we already have and taking good care of it, we have more energy for life and confidence in our capacity to be happy right now.

Thich Nhat Hanh has emphasized that a practitioner is somebody capable of generating joy and happiness at any moment and every moment that they want. I generate true happiness with mindfulness, concentration, and the right view that I am still alive. I am not a helpless child anymore. I am not a victim anymore. I can take care of myself. I can be with what was, what is, and what will be. I have people who care about me. I can give a voice to my suffering, get help, and transform it. These are right views, which bring the greatest happiness of all.

CHAPTER 10

True Love

We often use the word "love" to mean a desire to possess or consume something ("I love pizza!" "I love hot dogs!" "I love chocolate!" "I love you!"), but the way we speak about love in our culture shows that we don't really know what love entails. True love is healing. Sexual desire without love and respect is inevitably harmful. To heal trauma, we need to have the right understanding of love, and following the third mindfulness training of True Love helps us discern the difference between actions that cause us happiness and those that cause us suffering.

True Love begins with oneself. We must learn to be our own soul mates—remembering, knowing, and cherishing ourselves. When we are able to be a soul mate to ourselves, naturally we become a soul mate to others. Through the power of affinity, we will attract people who have respect and dignity for themselves, so they can love, accept, and respect us. This gift of true love must be mutual.

The Third Mindfulness Training: True Love

Aware of the suffering caused by sexual misconduct, I am committed to cultivating responsibility and learning ways to protect the safety and integrity of individuals, couples, families, and society. Knowing that sexual desire is not love, and that sexual activity motivated by craving

always harms myself as well as others, I am determined not to engage in sexual relations without true love and a deep, long-term commitment made known to my family and friends. I will do everything in my power to protect children from sexual abuse and to prevent couples and families from being broken by sexual misconduct. Seeing that body and mind are one, I am committed to learning appropriate ways to take care of my sexual energy and cultivating loving kindness, compassion, joy, and inclusiveness—which are the four basic elements of true love—for my greater happiness and the greater happiness of others. Practicing true love, we know that we will continue beautifully into the future.

The Four Basic Elements of True Love taught by the Buddha

1. Loving Kindness
2. Compassion
3. Joy
4. Inclusiveness

According to Thich Nhat Hanh, unless all four elements are there, we cannot say that true love is present. Practicing true love helps us have relationships that lead to healing instead of further traumas.

The third mindfulness training also asserts the importance of protecting children from sexual abuse. As we've seen, many victims of sexual abuse become perpetrators or enablers of abuse, knowingly or unknowingly. With this understanding, we learn to heal ourselves so that we do not repeat the cycle of abuse, recognizing the unhealthy and maladaptive signs and symptoms in ourselves and others and intervening appropriately.

Sexual Misconduct in Society

Child marriage. Female mutilation. Female sacrifice. Child trafficking. Child slavery. Child pornography. Adult pornography. Prostitution. Incest. Rape. Molestation. Sexual assault. Sexual harassment, sexual exploitation.... Sexual abuse has been so prevalent in all societies since the beginning of human evolution that it is a primary fabric of suffering in the world. Through our interconnectedness, sexual trauma is embedded deeply in every one of us!

In Buddhism, craving, anger, and ignorance are the three main mental poisons that generate and perpetuate suffering in the individual and the collective. The Buddha also taught that sexual energy, breath energy, and spiritual energy interrelate, one transforming into and affecting the other. Therefore, it is essential that practitioners learn to to channel sexual energy into the breath and spiritual energy for our own protection and freedom.

The fifth mindfulness training of Mindful Consumption via the six sense organs is supportive of true love. For example, many people nowadays consume pornography. They may start out of curiosity or to "escape," a word frequently used by our youth nowadays. They use electronic devices, the internet, movies, pornography, drugs, etc. to escape boredom, or difficult relationships and situations. Stress is the first arrow, desperation for escape is the second arrow, and unhealthy consumption compounds the suffering further. True Happiness, the second mindfulness training, has a direct causal effect on the third mindfulness training, True Love. Taking care of our three energies—sexual, breath, and spirit—through mindful consumption ensures that our sexual energy is balanced, healthy, and wholesome. Sex is not true love, and true love does not just entail sex. It may involve sexual interaction, but the six elements of True Love must be present as well. As I wrote in my book *Mindfulness as Medicine*, True Love always includes the right view of interbeing, healing, friendship, joy, respect, and trust. True Love should bring joy, not insecurity, confusion, doubt, or suffering.

Repetitive Cycles of Trauma in Adult Life

Keeping to the third mindfulness training also helps prevent couples and families from being broken by sexual misconduct. Many of us get involved in extramarital affairs because we are lonely and unhappy. Unable to take care of problems in ourselves and in our relationship, when we see someone coming along who seems empathetic, we grab on to that person like a lifesaver. Among reasons for having an affair, it is common to hear, "I feel alive again when I am with this new person."

The truth is, we can be on our best behavior in the beginning of a new romantic relationship, but once we feel comfortable in it we naturally return to our old ways. We will treat the new person the same way we have been treating our former spouse or partner, trapped in a Groundhog Day of our unconscious behaviors, endlessly repeating our grave mistakes and causing untold damage to the new person as well as to our original spouses and our children.

We try to escape from our problems by looking for something new, but we usually end up in a more serious dilemma. Sometimes the new person presents us with an even more complex set of issues than our previous partner. Ultimately, wherever we go, there we are. There is no escape from ourselves, our habits and destructive patterns; like a whiteboard eraser tainted with different colors, we keep bringing our past with us to new boards. If we do not know how to transform our wrong views, unskillful speech, and unhealthy behaviors, we repeat our pain and hurt in every relationship we go into, as if we are just marrying the same person again.

The example I often give is of my last foster dad. He was married to his sixth wife when my brother and I came to live with the family. He was cynical and sarcastic in his speech toward his wife; somewhat less so toward us. After I went to college, he got a divorce and married his seventh wife. I believe that he only stopped at the seventh wife because he got too old and sick to get married again. He never learned. Again, wherever you go, there you are.

Those of us who are in long-term relationships would do well to remember the third mindfulness training that "sexual desire is not love, and that sexual activity motivated by craving always harms myself as well as others." Sex should be consensual and pleasurable for both partners, an expression of love. Not infrequently, one person in a relationship will not feel "in the mood" for sex, but they will yield to their partner out of obligation or duty. Sad but true, sex is an obligation and duty in many relationships, including marriages. When women are in our perimenopause stage, which can take place up to ten years before menopause, our hormone levels drop quite dramatically, which can affect our general mood as well as our libido. Additionally, vaginal dryness and tightness can cause pain during sex. Many of us wish to sleep alone in our own rooms, on our own beds. This wish should be honored and respected. Instead of focusing on sex as the only way for intimacy, partners and spouses can help each other find ways to express our sensuality. Remember that even when our body is no longer fueled with sexual desire, our needs for meaningful companionship, attention, affection and love will always remain. We can embark on a spiritual journey together, which helps us rediscover ourselves and each other at deeper levels.

How to Not Be a Heartbreaker

One day at the end of a retreat during a teaching tour for young people in Seattle, a handsome young man approached me to request a private consultation. On the final morning of our retreats, participants always have an opportunity to take the Five Mindfulness Trainings in a ceremony with the whole community. "I wanted to talk to you yesterday, but I hesitated," he said. "I know this is my last chance today, so please give me some time." I sat down with him right then and there. His name was Ramón.

"I'm gay, and I admit I've had numerous irresponsible sexual encounters. I know a lot of people say gay people are hypersexual, and actually I did enjoy having an active sex life before coming here. So, this morning when I knelt to receive the Five Mindfulness Trainings, I really hesitated when it came to the third training of True Love. I wasn't sure if I should take the training or not because I know I won't be able to keep it. I want to ask you: How I can practice this training? I do not even know if I can practice True Love with the many sexual partners I currently have. Is it possible for me to practice true love?"

It turned out to be a long, profound conversation. First of all, I shared my thought that it was not because he was gay that he was more sexually active than the rest of the people he knew. Generally speaking, men may be more sexually preoccupied than women, because women ovulate only once a month, while men produce millions of sperm daily, and men's hormonal cycles fluctuate daily instead of monthly. In medical school I learned of a study showing that men think about sex every seven minutes! The male students seemed to agree, but the women in the class thought that was too often. I told Ramón that I had asked my brother if it was true that men think about sex once every seven minutes. He'd said, "No." A second later he added, "Much more often than that!"

"Seriously? What do you do about it?" I'd asked my brother incredulously.

"Most of the time I don't do anything about it, but sometimes I do something about it." That was my brother's answer, and Ramón agreed it was essentially his experience too.

Men, women, nonbinary folks, heterosexual, homosexual, bisexual, pansexual, or asexual, different people have different levels of sexual energy, depending on our genetic background, our culture, our environment, our previous sexual experiences, and our life choices. Our inherited sexual energy largely determines our own sexual energy. How we water it via our senses—through our eyes, ears, nose, mouth, body, and thoughts—will affect the strength of the craving and the manifestation of our sexual behaviors, balanced or not.

So, I shared with Ramón about mindful consumption and the Four Diligences of inviting and watering only wholesome seeds and not the unwholesome seeds.

He said, "Sister, I can see that my father was hypersexual, because he had two wives and several mistresses. Actually, both my parents were sexually active outside their marriage. So, I now see that some of my more reckless sexual choices had more to do with my conditioning and maybe genetics than because I am a gay man." Being hypersexual is learned behavior, but it also has a genetic component.

"Many people have multiple sexual partners throughout their life," I told him. "Very young people—from middle school or even younger—may already begin to have sexual encounters. These encounters can be careless and traumatic. Sex is just a game and a habit. The more you have sex without love, the less you believe in the existence of True Love, and you can't ever be truly happy.

"What do you seek, really? Have you had deep, long-lasting satisfaction through these experiences?" I asked Ramón.

"No, no, I feel a void afterward," he replied. "I still have to face myself and all this stress afterward, but I didn't know another way to connect. I saw casual sex being practiced by many people, and I just threw myself into it."

"Do you think about the effect you may be having on others? Even though you think it's enjoyable to have many partners, are you sure all your partners feel the same? Do you talk together about your emotions?" I shared with him what I had personally gone through with my uncle, and what happens when we mismanage our sexual energy, becoming abusers to ourselves and others. "My uncle was exposed to sex very early when he ran away from home as a young teenager, living on the street and getting involved in gang activities, including sex. It became a pattern for him. So even though he was normally a gentle person, he was secretly a sex addict, molesting me, and then, I later found out, my other female cousins."

As I was sharing with Ramón about my uncle, at some point tears began rolling down my cheeks. He too cried, and with loving tenderness, he dabbed at my tears and wiped them away. He exclaimed, "Sister D, I'm coming to realize that I have caused suffering to so many people! And, I didn't think it was related, but I was also molested as a child. I now see there is a connection.

"Sister D, I really understand now," he added. "I see a way to take care of myself from now on. When I look back, I realize I have caused a lot of people a lot of suffering, even if we were all consenting adults, and I never want to do that again. I certainly never want to hurt somebody like your uncle has hurt you."

Ramón spoke without shame or self-hatred, but with compassion for himself and for others. This young man saw the way out! It was clear that our conversation had changed his view and his approach to sexual relationships, right there and then. It was as if something clicked, an insight opened for him, and he was forever transformed. It was the shattering of a long-held belief and wrong view, freeing him from his own imprisonment of thinking that being an attractive man was equated with being hypersexual. He understood that True Love would include the right view of interbeing and would bring about healing, deep friendship, respect, trust, and confidence in his relationships.

If this young man could transform, he would save so many lives, because he was young, handsome, educated, and attractive—a heartbreaker, and proud to be one. Now he was determined to be a heart-protector instead.

Compulsive Sexuality Is Not True Love

Ramón also asked, "I have read that we need to masturbate because otherwise our fluids are stored in the body and it's unhealthy. Is this true?" This idea of "needing" to be sexual at all times for health reasons is a very common misconception among laypeople.

When I was doing volunteer work during medical school with incarcerated youth at San Francisco Youth Guidance Center, I frequently heard young men say, "If I don't jerk off, I'll turn green." In the seminal fluid that men produce daily, there are not only sperm but also calcium, glucose, and other nutrients to nourish the sperm. With excessive masturbation, the seminal fluid is continually used up, and the body responds by making more of it, using up the calcium, glucose, and other nutrients in the body. It is literally the energy and life force that are drained away. Worse yet, the mind can become obsessed with sexual thoughts. Instead of being present when working, or spending time with our family, we can become trapped in sexual mental consumption, which is drastically consuming and draining. The truth is, if we do not masturbate, the body will reabsorb any excess seminal fluid.

Sexual fantasies, dreams, and nocturnal emissions are normal physiological processes of the body, so they are nothing to be alarmed by or ashamed of. The practice is to simply recognize, breathe, and relax the sexual thoughts and physical sensations. Excessive consumption of sexual images and thoughts, on the other hand, can water the seeds of sexual craving, impelling us to masturbate and seek inappropriate, unhealthy sexual encounters to satisfy it. Drowning in a quagmire of lust, the consumer becomes consumed by it.

Drama Is Trauma

From my interactions with women of all ages and backgrounds over the years, as a doctor and then as a nun, I have learned that in addition to pleasure and affection, most of us look for acceptance, understanding, and companionship in relationships. Men also long for this: a person who knows you and accepts you as you are, who is there for you through thick and thin. A soul mate. Sadly, many of us end up settling for sex. It is the quickest way to feel intimacy, but it is only physical intimacy, and afterward we may feel awkward, restless, dissatisfied, and disappointed. Yet, like fireflies, we seek "love" from one person and then the next, subjecting our body and mind to trauma over and over again. Every sexual experience is registered and deposited, etched into our body and store consciousness, and the more careless or unhappy our sexual relationships are, the more cynical we become, and the less we believe in True Love. If a person does not believe in the existence of True Love, they cannot ever be happy.

Many young girls seeking acceptance and affection are at risk for sexual trauma. I have met young girls of sixteen or seventeen years old who have already had many boyfriends. Their mothers might be divorced or never married and might have had one boyfriend after another. Growing up seeing their mothers with many partners, they also entered sexual relationships very early, as young as ten, eleven, or twelve. Some girls have confided in me, "I've never been out of a relationship in my life." In the search for love and acceptance, they don't find it, but they put their bodies through sexual encounters that are at best mindless, but sometimes full of humiliation, pain, and sadness— drama. Dramas are traumas.

We are drawn to dramas. That's why soap operas and highly dramatic television shows are so popular. Korean dramas could make me cry from beginning to end, and yet I have to restrain myself from watching them at all! We are drawn to them. To learn to not be drawn into dramas, not to thrive on them, is actually an act of great compassion toward ourselves. It's harder than we think! People say "I don't want to suffer," but if we look at the way we consume with our eyes, ears, nose, mouth, body, and thoughts, we recognize that we feed our suffering all the time in all the different ways, because we're addicted to it. Dramas and suffering may be all that we know about relationships from our own lives, from our family life, and from society as a whole.

Love Is Healing

One of my mentees, Remy, a twenty-one-year-old woman who had experienced serious physical and sexual abuse in her childhood, was diagnosed with severe depression and anxiety in her early teens. She suffered from mental agony and before I met her, she resorted frequently to cutting and hair-pulling and thought constantly of suicide. By learning to meditate and consciously practicing the elements of true love with herself at the age of twenty-one, she has gradually learned to cherish and "reparent" herself.

Since we cannot meet in person at present, we continue to stay in touch via email. This is a message she sent to me recently:

> The wounds on my arms for many years have now healed. Isn't it a miracle, my dear Sister D? I kept thinking that those cuts would leave great ugly scars on my arms. But in the end, they have healed, and I have not caused any newer wounds.
>
> Every time I take a shower, I use the time to wash and massage my body lovingly and talk to myself, to my own spirit. Today I said, "I have made progress in taking better care of you, haven't I? Have your wounds healed? My darling spirit, I wish I could see your injuries the way I can see the scratches and cuts on my arms. But it is alright, I have strong faith that in the end, you too will heal, and even if you leave behind some little scars, that's okay too. Nothing is lost. I apologize to you, and I love you very much."
>
> I don't know why, but when I inquire about my own well-being like that, especially in asking my spirit, "Have your wounds healed?" my heart feels soothed and freer. It is true that attention and love bring healing, and healing is love, just like you have shared with me.

I converse with my spirit like I would to a young sister, a friend, and sometimes I speak like a mother. Perhaps sympathy and love are the best medicine for my spirit at this point. Sister D. you always remind me to say loving words to myself daily. It is true that I have caused myself to suffer so many times. Those people in the past caused suffering to my body, and then unknowingly I caused my body to suffer a second time. So, I am practicing correcting my ways, like the habit of pulling my hair, so I don't damage my body and my spirit anymore.

Looking at the new hair sprouting from my bald spots, I feel a lot of sorrow and regret. Anxiety and stress occasionally still cause me not to be able to stop pulling at my hair completely.

I do believe in what you have shared with me, that when my sadness and pain have healed, the habit of hurting myself will vanish automatically. Perhaps sometimes it will resurface, but I will be patient with myself. I should not think too much, and focus on the present, on my practice and all the love surrounding me.

These past few days, I was thinking too much again, so I got lost in the past and caused myself sadness. Thankfully, I became aware of it early, so nothing happened to me. I have gotten lost many times, so I have some experience in finding the way out. The experience also comes from the practice and from what Thay and you have shared with me. Now that I have the path, I do not need to be afraid anymore.

Please rest assured about me. I promise that I will not disappoint you.

Remy

CHAPTER 11

Loving Speech and Deep Listening

The fourth mindfulness training on Loving Speech and Deep Listening is for ourselves, first and foremost. In sitting meditation, we are practicing deep listening to ourselves, to our inner child. Practicing loving speech, we say to ourselves, "It's okay, I'm here for you. Please help me to understand you."

I have learned to tell myself "I love you" a hundred times a day. When I wake up, before I go to sleep, in the bathroom, while I am waiting for somebody, whenever I have pain. I say, "I love you" and "It's okay." In that way, I am training myself to be keenly aware of myself, truly present, listening deeply and responding lovingly toward myself. Only by expressing love toward ourselves first can we wholeheartedly offer loving speech and deep listening to other people.

The Fourth Mindfulness Training: Loving Speech and Deep Listening

Aware of the suffering caused by unmindful speech and the inability to listen to others, I am committed to cultivating loving speech and compassionate listening, in order to relieve suffering and to promote reconciliation and peace in myself and among other people, ethnic and religious groups, and nations. Knowing that words can create happiness or suffering, I am committed to speaking truthfully using words that inspire confidence, joy, and hope. When anger is manifesting in me, I am determined not to speak. I will practice mindful breathing and walking in order to recognize and to look deeply into my anger. I know that the roots of anger can be found in my wrong perceptions and lack of understanding of the suffering in myself and in the other person. I will speak and listen in a way that can help myself and the other person to transform suffering and see the way out of difficult situations. I am determined not to spread news that I do not know to be certain and not to utter words that can cause division or discord. I will practice Right Diligence to nourish my capacity for understanding, love, joy, and inclusiveness, and gradually transform anger, violence, and fear that lie deep in my consciousness.

Speaking Lovingly Is a Learned Skill

If we had a rough time growing up, it's only natural that we have to relearn how to communicate well with ourselves and others, without bringing in our habits from the past. There was a young monastic sister who'd had a lot of suffering in her childhood and teenage years, so she could be quite harsh and brusque to the other sisters in her speech and actions. Yet she was so loving and tenderhearted toward animals. One time, she rescued a little baby bird that had fallen out of its nest and tended to it until it was strong enough to fly away. One day, I said to her jokingly, but seriously too, "You know, if you treated us the way you treat the cats and the birds, we'd be very happy." She took my words to heart and made an effort to change. She began speaking more gently to us after that, and soon enough found that people responded to her in kind.

If we are able to love something nonhuman, say a bird or an animal, then we can learn to translate that love toward ourselves, and then slowly toward others. This is why spending time with pets and connecting with nature can make a big difference to trauma survivors.

Remy, the young woman in chapter 10, had been on high doses of antidepressants and anxiolytics for many years, which did not prevent her from cutting herself and harming herself in several ways. Remy's most visible anxiety symptom was hair-pulling. The bald spots on her scalp were so large they looked like burn scars, which she disguised by strategically pinning her hair over them. As a child, Remy had been subjected to severe abuse by her babysitter.

Remy wrote this letter to me soon after one of our conversations:

Dear Sister D,

Even though my habit of pulling on my hair has decreased, when I am stressed, I cannot stop pulling my hair completely. There are times when I cannot control it at all, so I join my palms together to stop myself. Still, at other times I succumb to the habit.

Recently, I discovered that besides the feeling of satisfaction I get from hair pulling, there is also this thought coming up from the depths of my mind that having hair is unlucky, and I want to uproot all of that unluckiness so my heart can be lighter. Logically, I know it doesn't make sense, but when I am stressed, I lose my control.

I asked myself where this belief about "unlucky" hair came from. Both of my parents like their girls to grow long hair. My saddest memory relating to my hair had to do with my babysitter, who yanked on my hair and poured hot water on my head, but she did not refer to my hair as "unlucky." I recall that when she was combing my hair, she would pull it backward, causing my scalp to bleed at times. So, I am not sure whether I pull on my hair because I am stressed or because of this unpleasant past.

Each time that image of my babysitter arose, I just wanted to block it out and not look deeply into the cause of my hair pulling anymore. Yet, I really want to stop this habit. Perhaps I need more time to work on it. I keep remembering what you taught me, that each strand of my hair also needs my love, just like I need love. Dear Sister, I tell myself I love my hair and I do want to heal.

I advised Remy to scan her body often and to give thanks to each part; to tell her body "I love you" several times a day; and to remember that each strand of her hair also needs her love, just like she needs love. While self-harm habits like hair pulling are hard to change, Remy's hair eventually did grow back, a sign that Remy's loving speech was able to undo at least some of the harm triggered by her trauma.

Every mindfulness training is a practice of true love, and loving speech and deep listening are trainings in giving and receiving and creating more love in the world. For example, walking mindfully, you can listen attentively to your steps and realize that when you have feelings of hatred or negativity, your steps are heavy, pounding on the Earth. We literally stamp our feet with anger and aggression on the earth. Think of soldiers and the sound of marching feet. On the other hand, your steps are gentle and quiet when you feel peaceful. Our steps faithfully reflect and manifest our emotions. With awareness of our anger, we intentionally practice walking meditation so that we are not pounding on the ground, not hurting our joints and body, and not rehearsing our suffering.

I like to quietly sing to myself fragments of Thich Nhat Hanh's poems as I walk. *The mind can go in a thousand directions, but on this path,*

I walk in peace. With each step a gentle wind blows. With each step a flower blooms. Or, I may hold in my mind as I walk, "Each step is peace," "Each step is healing," "Come back, come back to this moment." Thus, loving speech and deep listening can take place throughout the day. Deep listening to our own breathing patterns, our steps, the sensations in our body, our thoughts, our feelings, our views gives rise to a feeling of love. Whatever arises, we can say, "It's okay, we'll take care of it, one thing at a time," and affirm our self-love and compassion, remembering always, "I am here for you."

Denial and the Importance of Speaking Up

A social worker I met once told me that DENIAL stands for: Don't Even Know I Am Lying. That really stuck with me.

For victims of abuse, denial can be a self-protecting mechanism. Many people literally do not remember the incident or only have vague recollections or snapshots of it; in this case, the nervous system has automatically blocked out the experience for self-survival purposes. Or we may have varying degrees of awareness about what has taken place, but we immerse ourselves in work, relationships, or entertainment in order to not have to confront the trauma. Many families do not recognize the abuse that is taking place in their children because they are so preoccupied with their problems, or because they themselves were victims of abuse, and they cannot face this issue in their own children. Like Claire's mother in chapter 3, they unconsciously engage in a blanket of denial, desperate to cling to the thought, "This is not happening to me or to my family."

In addition to on the individual and family scale, we recognize that denial about misconduct is happening on a global scale. Just as the numbers of incidents of child abuse are large, so is the amount of denial. Different societies are at different points along the way in terms of openness to talking about sexual abuse. The worldwide #MeToo movement did a lot to break down taboos. When I was last in Vietnam, I was also relieved to see billboards on the streets asking people to report cases of child sexual abuse—a sign that even in relatively conservative Vietnamese society, people are courageously speaking up.

Some of us are confused about loving speech, thinking it means we should not say anything negative, ever. For example, the sentence in the fourth mindfulness training, "I am determined not to spread news that I do not know to be certain and not to utter words that can cause division or discord," could be misinterpreted as encouraging people to keep quiet about abuse because it causes the harm to surface, to be seen and addressed. For those in the family who are in denial, speaking about harm feels unbearably uncomfortable. "If we don't talk about it, it isn't true, and it doesn't exist" is how denial works. As we saw in the story of Claire in chapter 3, denial is ultimately very damaging to relationships. Indeed, we need to create a culture in which we can speak about harm in a way that is restorative to survivors. It may be helpful to remember the words of the fourth mindfulness training, "to speak truthfully using words that inspire confidence, joy, and hope."

Not addressing a harmful situation with appropriate action is also a form of denial. As we deny the gravity of a situation, we are lying to ourselves. We do not even know we are lying to ourselves, and it is most damaging because we block our own chance for calling out for help and receiving help when it's offered to us. People who use drugs or suffer from depression or anxiety may adamantly reject help and treatment because they do not see that they have a problem.

The harm of denial applies equally to perpetrators. Perpetrators of sexual abuse may in their own minds defend themselves with excuses such as, "She tempted me" or, "What I did wasn't that bad." My own uncle told me repeatedly, "Don't tell your mother. What we are doing is good for you."

May I Kiss You?

From my own practice and healing, I can now bring awareness to my own family—my niece, my brother, my sister-in-law, and her mother—so that they can also recognize and prevent abuse. They do not leave my young niece, Sunee, alone in the house or anywhere by herself with anyone outside the immediate family, even her cousins or her uncles.

I teach my niece, Sunee, that her body is her own. When she was a toddler, she was so precious and adorable to me, sometimes I just wanted to hug and kiss her all over! But children do not want to be kissed, except by people with whom they are very close, such as their mothers and fathers, and not necessarily even by them. Even though my niece is quite close to me, she doesn't kiss me often or allow me to kiss her. Even when I hug her, she turns her back to me. I see many children do this. One time I was overcome by affection and wanted to kiss her, so I gave her a kiss on her cheek. She screamed, "Don't do that! I don't like it!" I felt so hurt for a moment. I breathed, quieted myself, and then gently said to her, "I'm sorry. I am glad you told me that." From then on, I have always tried to remember to ask her permission to hug her or to kiss her instead of assuming my actions are okay for her.

One time, I asked her permission to kiss her, but she said no. Then she added, "But I can shake your hand." I laughed, "Yes, we definitely can shake hands." Then I told her she could tell other people the same thing if she didn't feel comfortable with their kisses.

I saw Sunee again a few days later, to go out to the park. She was removing her clothes and changing her outfit right in front of me; I wanted to say something to her, but I hesitated because I wasn't sure if she would understand. I gently asked her, "Do you know that your body is sacred?" She asked, "What is 'sacred' Chô Chô?" So, I explained to Sunee, "Sacred means your body is very special. It means that no one can touch your body without your permission." "Yeah," she said nonchalantly.

To test her understanding, I asked her what she would she say if someone wanted to kiss her. She answered, "No! You cannot kiss me, but ... you can shake my hand." I was so pleased because she still remembered our recent conversation.

Then I asked, "What do you say if someone wants to kiss your lips?" She answered clearly, "No!"

Then I pointed to her chest. She asserted with a *humph*, "No!" as she crossed her hands in front of her chest.

Then I pointed to her belly. She crossed in hands in front of her belly and said, "No!" even louder and more energetically.

I pointed to her genital area. She crossed her hands over it and shouted, "*No!*"

I was so pleased to see her confident responses. I added, "And if anyone tries to touch you without your permission, you can tell your parents, your grandma, or your teacher." I paused for a moment, trying to think of who else she could tell.

Lo and behold, Sunee declared affirmatively, "I'll tell my parents! I'll tell my grandma! I'll tell my teachers! I'll tell my friends! I'll tell everybody in the whole world! *Don't you dare to touch my body without my permission!*"

I burst out laughing, and tears were streaming down my face at the same time. I hadn't been sure if she would understand what I was trying to teach her, but she understood well beyond my tentative lesson. In that moment, the frightened and confused nine-year-old girl in me rejoiced with Sunee in chorus, "*Yes, I will tell everybody in the whole world! Don't you dare to touch my body without my permission!*"

A child will understand this message if we use their language. If we are close to them and we build trust, we can teach them that their bodies are sacred, precious, and to be respected, by themselves and by others. We can teach them that they have the right to say no loudly and with confidence to anything, and they have the right to know that nothing is wrong with them.

Children never have the intention of bringing any sort of abuse upon themselves, so we have to pay attention and believe a child whenever they report anything. They may not speak with absolute clarity, but may allude to their feelings, saying, "I'm not comfortable," "He's touching me there," "She's touching me there," "I have pain here," "I'm scared," or "He's chasing me in my dreams." We must tune in and tend to those comments immediately and skillfully with loving speech and deep listening. We must find out who is involved and how to protect the child from further harm, instead of questioning the child skeptically, because that will shut them down and they may never share something in that nature with us again. Expressing doubt to a child is to inflict another layer of trauma on them.

Listening to Children

To understand is to listen, and to listen is to understand. The rule of thumb is when you hear children in your life talking about any kind of conflict—verbal disagreement, physical fight, or harm done to their bodies or to another child's body—please stop what you are doing, sit down at their level, and listen to them.

- Express your desire to understand more about the incident.

- Gently encourage them to speak with questions like, "Tell me more." Children may not be able to articulate their feelings clearly, so you ask them specific questions like: "How does it feel in your body?" "Where do you feel it in your body? Can you point to where you are having that feeling?"

- If the child is not comfortable sharing more, don't press them. Discreetly and skillfully observe their physical appearance, their speech, their word choice, their moods and behaviors, and return to the topic afterward.

True Remorse Is Restorative

A good friend once shared with me that in the last moments of her mother's life, the dying woman was still waiting for her husband to acknowledge the deep wounds he had inflicted on her. During their marriage, her father had betrayed her mother, but he would never talk about it or apologize to her. At one point during the vigil, my friend pleaded with her father to go talk to her mother. He went into the room, looked at his wife's face, and said just two words: "I'm sorry." Her mother passed away within seconds after he left the room, finally able to let go.

Some of us are waiting for the other person to say "I'm sorry" all our lives. It is more important than we know. Right before I began medical school, I returned to Vietnam and confronted my uncle about his abuse for the first time. We had never talked about it; we had rarely even been in the same room since I had gone to live in the United States.

I was unsure how to start the conversation. We went to sit outdoors in an open field. I suddenly asked him, "Do you remember what you did to me? Why did you do that to me? I was just a child, while you were already a grown man, handsome, with many beautiful women pursuing you. Why?"

He broke down crying, and on his knees, he said in a wretched voice, "I am so sorry. I am so sorry. I was so stupid then!"

At that moment, my heart opened. Strangely, I found myself willing to forgive him. Perhaps it was to let go of the burden of hatred and aversion I had been carrying for so long. Of course, it took me many more years to learn how to heal and forgive myself, but after his apology I felt more comfortable being in the same room with him for the rest of the time I was at home visiting.

To express regret is crucial, because denial of the abuse prevents the situation from ever being repaired. When a perpetrator says "I did not do it. You must have imagined it," and denies or minimizes the harm, it is a second crime. Receiving an apology in our lifetimes may help take a huge brick out of our wall of suffering and allow in some light.

However, even if we do receive a heartfelt apology, we need to continue to take care of ourselves and—this is very important—not internalize the perpetrator of abuse within ourselves with negative self-talk. We may have a habit of *unloving* speech and *shallow* listening to ourselves! Frequently survivors of abuse feel stupid, worthless. Thus, every time you feel prone to telling yourself "You are stupid," instead try to say to yourself "I'm sorry," and express your wish to practice loving speech and deep listening with yourself. As well as gratitude toward others, we need to say thank you to ourselves, and thus we come out of our habit of unloving speech toward ourselves.

Speaking Truthfully Is Protective

In recent years, I found out that my uncle had molested two of my younger cousins *after* I had confronted him about the sexual abuse he had inflicted on me. One of these cousins became pregnant and gave birth to their child on the street. The child looked exactly like my uncle, who was her father as well as grand-uncle.

Rage and pain filled my heart when I found out about this. By that time, my uncle had been dead for many years, but many lives continued to be affected by him. Although I had never met my cousin, I felt her pain deeply and wanted to reach out to comfort her. I felt co-responsible for her suffering. When I visited Vietnam last year, I wrote my young cousin a short letter, saying,

> Our uncle caused you pain and injustice. In the end, he paid for it with his early death, burdened by illnesses. Please do not blame yourself. Take good care of your life. Take good care of your daughter. I love you.

My mother's older sister did not want to admit the abuses committed against my two younger cousins by my uncle, her own brother. My mother's second cousin was the one to tell me about it. In turn, I finally told her about my own abuse, and she wept and cried. She hugged me and kept crying, "I can't believe it! I'm so sorry!" I told her, "It's okay. I have healed. But I'm devastated to know that he continued to commit these crimes. I am so sorry too."

The family and the community *always* need to be told. It is the secrecy, shame, and taboo of talking about sexual misconduct that allow it to continue. Furthermore, sexual abuse can become habitual for the perpetrator if they do not get help. They usually repeat the abuse and have more than one victim. That is why we need to raise awareness to prevent them from hurting others and also so that the perpetrator can have an opportunity to heal before they cause any further suffering in the world.

Expressing Regret Is an Act of Courage

A Hollywood film producer once shared with me his concerns about the #MeToo movement. On the one hand, he held genuine respect for the women who spoke up, because he knew they were speaking the truth and the system was completely wrong. On the other hand, he had a fear that some women could be out to make money or take advantage of the outpouring of support for the movement.

"Say I put my arms around somebody's shoulder, genuinely being nice and friendly? What if they turn around and now say I was sexually harassing them?" he asked. "I don't even dare to ask a woman out for dinner anymore, because she might accuse me of sexually harassing her!"

He was so concerned about his predicament that I had to laugh and tease him a little. Then I told him that it was good that he was aware of the suffering women have been facing. Now he would have to do the work of being more sensitive and mindful of how he might be treating other people. He would need to become more conscious of his position of power, as a man and as a film producer.

Then, taking a more serious tone, I also advised him to look back to see if he might have crossed the line in some ways with some women. It would be healing if he could approach them now and apologize to them, saying, "I know now I was not always mindful, so if I have ever made you feel uncomfortable, please forgive me."

For a moment, he seemed to be moved by what I said, as he contemplated how expressing his regrets would free him from his burden of fear and anxiety. But then he felt afraid again that the women would use his apology as evidence to sue him!

Expressing regret for past actions takes real courage. It takes an attitude of caring more for the person you have harmed than for your own self-image. It may help to remember that the act of apology can be healing and empowering to both parties, and is a needed step on the path toward repairing damaged relationships and reconciling with those we have hurt. Practicing the training of loving speech and deep listening can help us find this courage.

CHAPTER 12

Nourishment and Healing

The fifth mindfulness training is on the subject of mindful consumption, and true to the spirit of interbeing, the one contains the all. The fifth training contains all the other four trainings.

Nourishment and Healing

Aware of the suffering caused by unmindful consumption, I am committed to cultivating good health, both physical and mental, for myself, my family, and my society, by practicing mindful eating, drinking, and consuming. I will practice looking deeply into how I consume the Four Kinds of Nutriments, namely edible foods, sense impressions, volition, and consciousness. I am determined not to gamble, or to use alcohol, drugs, or any other products which contain toxins, such as certain websites, electronic games, TV programs, films, magazines, books, and conversations. I will practice coming back to the present moment to be in touch with the refreshing, healing, and nourishing elements in me and around me, not letting regrets and sorrow drag me back into the past nor letting anxieties, fear, or craving pull me out of the present moment. I am determined not to try to cover up loneliness, anxiety, or other suffering by losing myself in consumption. I will contemplate interbeing and

> consume in a way that preserves peace, joy, and well-being
> in my body and consciousness, and in the collective body
> and consciousness of my family, my society, and the Earth.

Again, as with all the trainings, we first make sure we are applying this training in a way that is kind and expansive, not punitive or restricting. We relate the training of nourishing and healing to consumption in the broadest sense, especially the ingestion of our own thoughts, feelings, and perspectives.

We live in a consumer society, in which the things we turn to for comfort are marketed to us without our best interests in mind. While edible food is of course the basis of our existence (without food, the first of the Four Nutriments, our bodies cannot live), in trauma healing we need to be most mindful of our consumption through the senses and the mind. In particular, we should recognize that our use of social media and online interactions can be unwholesome and actually damaging to our ability to relate to others.

Some of our coping mechanisms since childhood or our teenage years may be self-destructive in the long-term. As a society, we need to teach ourselves and our children ways of being with what is. Our mindfulness practice is to be there for what is, not to escape from reality. To hold and embrace; to soothe, and then to investigate the situation and find a way out as soon as possible; this should be our practice. Not to let ourselves escape year after year.

Are You Addicted to Technology?

In my brother's family, I noticed how electronics were used to babysit my niece, Sunee, especially by her grandma. When Grandma needed to do some work, she would say, "Sunee, here's your iPad. Play with it." Or when they were going somewhere, Grandma would remind Sunee to bring her iPad. Sunee learned to distract and soothe herself with her iPad, without needing too much attention from adults.

This is the case for many children nowadays. You can just leave a child with a smartphone or tablet, and the child will sit still for five hours, instead of playing outside. Even when going out for a walk, parents bring devices to keep their children quiet. It is disturbing and sad to see a two-year-old sitting in a stroller in a park, eyes glued to the screen, without caring to look around.

Sometimes when I went to visit Sunee, she would look unhappy and frown at me because my arrival would interrupt her in the middle of playing a game on her iPad. Admittedly, I felt hurt by that, because it was not easy for me to leave the monastery to go see her, and I felt put out that she would prefer the company of her screen to that of her devoted aunt.

One day, when she was six years old, I couldn't help myself and I told Sunee, "You are addicted to electronics!" She asked me, "What does 'addicted' mean?" I explained, "It's when you cannot control yourself, when you keep going to it, and you're not even aware of it. It has control over you. That is addiction."

Ever since Sunee was a toddler, she would tell her dad, "Stop smoking, Daddy, stop smoking!" She was quite adamant and righteous about it, having heard her mother warning her father about how harmful tobacco is to the health. Not long after our conversation about addiction, one day she said to her dad: "Daddy, are you addicted to cigarettes, like I'm addicted to technology?" My brother laughed so hard! But I was very impressed by how she made the connection. Sunee saw the link, and it built up her empathy for her dad. Before that, she had wanted him to stop smoking, but she did not understand what that entailed. However, when she understood the idea of addiction and admitted that she too was addicted, to technology, she could understand her father better.

I notice a strong pattern among Vietnamese young people who were born or raised in the US, whom I meet in the course of teaching. They start to play games or watch movies at a very young age, given devices to be their babysitters. Being instantly entertained becomes a habit for them, and they feel out of sorts when they don't have access to the internet. I've met children who tell me they play electronics nine hours a day when they are out of school. They may stay on their devices even if they are in school, until two in the morning or later. Their parents are unaware of this because they are sleeping, and soon their parents can no longer stop them.

The brain continues to make new connections throughout childhood and trim off unused ones vigorously during the adolescent years. As they become dependent and addicted to their electronics, young people only receive input passively, and the devastating effect of this is that they develop only certain motor skills, while the rest of the brain is neglected. Their social skills also worsen with time. They lose communication with their parents because their parents seem boring compared to the virtual world. Friendships in middle and high school take place almost entirely online. Anyone who spends time with teens has seen how friends sitting next to each other text instead of looking at each other in the eyes and conversing directly.

Many parents, because they want their children to eat, bring food to the room so they can play and eat at the same time. Obesity, insomnia, lethargy, and poor school performance are prevalent symptoms among gamers and YouTubers. Children as young as eight years old on our retreats report that they have poor vision, neck pain, and back pain from playing on their devices! It is good to question why and how we have integrated electronic media so deeply into our lives, at such a deep cost. Our whole culture has become centered around electronic communication very rapidly in the past few decades, and those of us who value life off-screen may feel like members of a defiant minority.

Electronic Dependency as a Coping Mechanism

I hear teenagers using the word "escape" frequently. Electronic dependency is a negative coping mechanism for escape—escape your difficulties, escape your parents, escape the stress of school, escape responsibilities. When you play games, watch movies, or get engrossed in social media, your reward center is stimulated, releasing endorphins, the feel-good hormone. Like the character of Gifty, a neuroscience PhD candidate in Yaa Gyasi's novel *Transcendent Kingdom*, researchers have found that mice will keep pressing the lever to give themselves addictive drugs once they discover that it makes them feel good. They keep pressing until they become exhausted. Some even die. They cease eating and drinking and keep pressing the lever instead, just to feel good.

Similarly, we find comfort and escape in consuming media via our electronic devices—not only young people but all of us. It is the abnormal norm now. Adults and working professionals can also become dysfunctional when we spend many hours doing computer/internet/video game activities. Symptoms to internet addiction include:

- changes in mood,
- preoccupation with the internet and digital media,
- the inability to control the amount of time spent interfacing with digital technology,

- the need for more time or a new game to achieve a desired mood,
- withdrawal symptoms when not engaged,
- a continuation of the behavior despite family conflict,
- a diminishing social life, and
- adverse work or academic consequences.*

The World Health Organization has formally acknowledged internet addiction as a globally significant public health threat to people of all ages. There are hospitals and clinics in the US that admit people who have internet addiction as inpatients to receive medication and therapy.

For trauma survivors, electronic usage can be a quick and effective way to escape the waves of suffering that keep surfacing in our minds. Unfortunately, the more we use the mechanism of escape and suppression instead of stopping and facing our problems, the more relentless and powerful those waves become. Every aspect of our lives may be affected and become dysfunctional.

I once counseled Sylvie, who had lost her boyfriend when she was seventeen years old. Her mother encouraged her to date another person, but that relationship only depressed her and caused her revulsion. Over the last fifteen years, she had become dependent on online gaming, which was her only social life. Her eating habits and sleep-wake pattern became completely dysfunctional, which caused her to look underdeveloped for her age, and I suspected anorexia. She has to wear a wig because her hair cannot grow. Even the growth of her nails became stunted, so that she needs to wear artificial nails.

---

* "Internet Addiction: A Brief Summary of Research and Practice," Hilarie Cash, Cosette D. Rae, Ann H. Steel, and Alexander Winkler, The National Center for Biotechnology Information, www.ncbi.nlm.nih.gov/pmc/articles/PMC3480687/.

Although she was quite reserved and skeptical at first, gradually she was able to openly express her loss and pain. She also recognized the negative coping mechanisms that she had developed over the years and was able, with the Five Mindfulness Trainings, to unwind her habits and establish a future in which she could experience joy offline. In her last consultation with me, she said, "I hope that in my life, I am able to help even just one person." I told her that the one person who deserves her help and her love is herself. As we hugged each other at the end, she whispered to me, "Finally, somebody understands!"

A Source of Trauma in Itself

In other people I have met, dependence on electronic devices for social and emotional support may have started without a specific underlying trauma, but then the addiction becomes traumatic in itself. For example, many children may not have familial trauma, but they are trained to use electronics for finding rewards and comfort. Repeated reward-seeking behaviors become habits and, worse yet, addictions. As a result, when you run into difficulties in your teenage and adult lives, you may resort to your electronic friends to escape stress, tension, and pain, instead of taking care of your issues in a mindful way. Consequently, electronic dependency may first become a negative coping mechanism, a habit developed at an early age, and then a cause of unhappy outcomes later in life.

Pierre, the husband of my best friend from college, is a self-professed gaming addict. They have been married over twenty years, and every day he would come home from work and play video games until two or three in the morning. My friend had to be the main caretaker of their children. Recently, she told me that Pierre is so morbidly obese now, in his forties, that if he were to vacuum the house as she requested, afterward he'd be in bed for two days because of back pain. "So, I might as well just do the housework so he doesn't lose his job after too many sick days," she said. His gaming is a source of trauma in itself, causing ill-health in himself, loneliness in the spouse, stress in the relationship, and estrangement from his children.

I know a young man who was brilliant in high school, and he could get away with playing video games right after school and into the night. Once in college as an engineering major, he struggled with insomnia, still playing games and unable to focus on his schooling. As a result, he could not pass his courses and dropped out of his chosen path, wrapped in disappointment and self-loathing.

There is a stereotype that young men are the most affected by media overconsumption, but in fact, girls and young women also play a lot of video games, or they watch hours and hours of dramas, anime, action movies, or whatever fits their personality and culture. We might think this kind of entertainment is harmless taken in moderation, but we need to remember that the dramas out there may become our own life dramas—because everything we are exposed to will be deposited into our consciousness, influencing our worldview and triggering us to think, speak, and behave accordingly.

Either way, whether you have pre-existing trauma or not, excessive electronic usage is a kind of suffering. The addiction itself is traumatic. People feel engaged and alive only while they are online, and they feel zombie-like, numb, and lost in the real world. Social isolation can lead to antisocial behaviors, depression, and self-harm.

If we are members of a non-dominant social group, the risk of trauma is even higher, no matter how well our parents try to trauma-proof our environment. Two older teen boys came to the monastery family retreat last summer. They sat by their tent, immobile, their faces startlingly similar with the same catatonic, vacant stare. Their parents had to beg them to attend at least one activity a day. When I held one of the brothers' hands during a circle, it was like holding a dry stick, stiff and lifeless. When I let go of his hand, it just stayed there, suspended in midair.

Their parents were immigrants, working hard outside of the home most of the day, and since an early age they had left their kids home alone with just their electronic devices after school. The parents felt estranged from their boys and were at a loss as to how to reconnect with them. They felt they had sacrificed so much to give their children a better life, without seeing that it was at the cost of the mental health of the entire family. Now the parents were worried that their children wouldn't be able to finish school, get a job, have a family, and live "a normal American life," which they had worked so hard for their children to have. Over the course of the retreat, the parents came to see that they needed to spend time with their children and not let them continue to be traumatized by neglect.

Electronic Liberators

At our annual teen retreats, we request that teenagers let go of their devices for the week, so that they can be fully present for the retreat and for each other. We ask them to hand in their phones and other electronic gadgets to our monastic brothers and sisters, whom we call our monastic "electronic liberators." When the teens first arrive, initially there is a huge resistance to this idea, but by the end of the retreat they almost all report having made closer connections with each other and experiencing life at a deeper and more peaceful level, and they unanimously approve of continuing this policy!

Working with teenagers, we try to raise awareness in them and engage their critical thinking by asking them questions such as:

- Are you using your phone or is your phone using you?
- Are you truly making a connection with those you associate with via social media?
- Are you aware of the effects social media has on you?
- What do you think are the intentions of people who are constantly advertising new applications and the newest devices?

With social media, you may feel so connected to people on the other side of the world, but to those people who are nearest to you, you may have become distant and disassociated. And the connections you do have with people far away are likely superficial. For example, people tend to pose only nice pictures and special events on TikTok or Facebook or Snapchat, showing off their great lives. Everybody looks great. Everybody looks happy! You may feel depressed afterward because you feel your life is so boring and bleak by comparison.

The truth is that people only post great moments. They don't dine at restaurants like that all the time. They may argue before and after the meal, or they may be busy doing selfies and posting pictures instead of talking to each other. Nobody knows that. No one posts that. Social media is extremely misleading. The glamour takes place in only a split second, and the rest of the time people are dealing with their life challenges and dramas. Do we ever think about that? In their hunger for more authentic connection, the current teen generation "Z" purposely posts "ugly" photos of themselves and "real" moments from their lives, but market forces are such that even authenticity can become a commodity on social media, to be ranked, rated, and sold.

Therefore, we need to reach out to young people and raise their awareness about the effects that electronic abuse can have on their physical, mental, and intellectual development. Parents, I encourage you to make more time to be with your children. Don't use electronics as a babysitter, or a substitute for you. A device cannot replace your love, your attention, your conversation, your daily interaction with your children.

Adults need to reflect on our own use and acknowledge how dependent we are on electronics. For example, when we have a spare moment, we automatically get out our phones. Recognize that. Breathe and put it down. It has become second nature now to hold on to an electronic gadget, surfing for news or watching videos on YouTube in our precious "free time." Nowadays when I go to the airport or public places, I see people with their eyes glued to screens, drawn outwardly away from themselves. Like our animal ancestors, we all have a great capacity to be aware of the outside the way a cat is aware of the mouse. However, the capacity to be aware of our own bodily movements and of our own thoughts and feelings—be it fear, anticipation, joy, or peace—has developed more recently in humans through evolution. Unfortunately, if we are on autopilot most of the time, then we are not cultivating further our endowed capacity for self-awareness. We use our body all day long, but we are hardly aware of it. We're like those drivers who use their vehicles without paying attention to rumbling warning sounds, faltering parts, or emptying gas tanks.

We keep saying that we don't have enough time. Yet if we look at how we spend our time, we will see that we waste a lot of energy. A lot of our time and energy leaks out through social media, with the hope of getting social acknowledgment, recognition, and comfort—but ultimately we inevitably find that it's not as satisfying or long-lasting as in-person interaction. Often, we use social media only as a way of escaping our own life. Before, people used drugs or alcohol; now they use electronics. People think it's harmless, but in the end it may be even more harmful than alcohol or drugs. The dopamine hits we get from social media are drugs in themselves, and they pervade every aspect of our life. Electronic addiction is currently a socially acceptable addiction.

The solution is to have more awareness. Only awareness will bring change. We need to connect with each other and share our aspirations for our human family, so that we may stop over-consuming on all levels and lead happy lives.

I've often talked to my niece about electronic addictions and their devastating effects on young people, to which I have been witness. I tell her: "You have a brilliant mind. I really want you to take care of your mind. It would break my heart to see you become sick, losing your intelligence, your wittiness, your bright personality. Don't zone out and become a zombie! Even though you are young, I trust that you understand my concerns. You need to protect your brain, so that it can develop in the healthiest way possible."

Amazingly, after one of these talks, when her mother took her iPad away, Sunee did not complain. Since then, she has been spending much less time on electronics, because she understands the link between consumption, her mind, and her mood.

The Harm of Pornography

In one Dharma sharing group at a retreat, a teen boy shared that he felt his life was so dull, he thought about death all the time. His words moved the other young people in the group. After the group ended, he stayed behind and said, "Sister D, can I talk to you?"

I immediately sat down with him. He said, "There's something I want to share with you privately, because I couldn't share it with everybody. I have been watching a lot of pornography, all the time, and it made me feel really sick. At some point, I realized that I should stop, but I couldn't. Being at this retreat the last few days, I've had no access to porn and I feel great. I really don't want to go back to it."

I talked with him about the different practices of self-care and true love, as described earlier in this book. "Instead of viewing women as sexual objects, you could also cultivate empathy and compassion for them," I said. "The women you've seen on your screen are actually real people—somebody's mothers, sisters, daughters, grandchildren. They could be your own sisters or cousins." He nodded in acknowledgment. "I can now see that sexual craving doesn't bring me real happiness, but it takes away my energy and waters the 'negative seeds' in me."

Children have easy access to the internet, and there is no end to it. Sexual images are just a few clicks away, and people have become so desensitized to the consumption of pornography that the industry is creating more and more extreme forms to hold the interest of the marketplace. Children are curious. Adults are curious. The more we watch, the more we want to watch. It becomes an addiction before we know it, and as with any compulsive behavior, it requires strong insight to end it and make a commitment to mindful consumption.

Awareness about this issue needs to be raised. Our conscience as a society may become numb to what is right, what is wrong, and what is proper. One large subsection of online pornography is incest, such as scenarios of sex with family members, with subjects like "Sexy Stepsister" or "Sexy Stepdaughter." Sadly, the prevalence of this kind of pornography reflects our store consciousness of taboo topics, full of negative seeds we do not want to water in regular society, yet allow to proliferate with far-reaching effects on the social and individual psyche.

Pornography involving children is sadly also common. Farrah, a friend now in her forties, shared with me that the youngest members of her large extended family—herself, her siblings, and her cousins— had all been objects of child pornography, organized by her aunts and uncles. Family gatherings at Christmas and other holidays and vacations became times for them to conduct filming. It was frightening, bewildering, but they did not disclose it to their parents right away.

She said, "It's amazing how I was only eleven years old, and I was dressed all in skimpy clothing, and yet my mother never questioned me about it. My cousins were dressed up like that too. I guess if you look at clothes put out for children by major fashion chains, they tend to be sexy, so Mom and Dad didn't notice much difference."

All the children became hypersexual. Cousins sat on each other's laps, touching each other in a sexual way whenever they got together. This went on until Farrah's younger sister had a psychotic breakdown after one of their family gathering-filming sessions. Coming back to their own home, the child blurted everything out, the obscene and profane, finally getting their parents' attention. Farrah's parents completely disowned the rest of the family, moved away, and cut all family ties to this day.

Farrah reported that her cousins became highly promiscuous later in life and were unable to have normal relationships or healthy lives because they were all so deeply affected by this. Thankfully, she found ways to heal herself through mindfulness, yoga, therapy, and spiritual practices. By nourishing herself with wholesome activities, thoughts, and relationships, today Farrah is radiant, loving, and healthy in body and mind, an embodiment of the teaching, "Be beautiful, be yourself."

In another retreat, while we were discussing the Five Mindfulness Trainings, a recently married young man confessed that he had never questioned his viewing pornography until we began talking about the fifth training of Mindful Consumption. He had watched pornographic videos online before he got married, and he continued to watch them afterward too. He said, "The discussion today makes me wonder how my wife would feel about it. I've never asked her!" I encouraged him to ask his wife how she felt about his viewing pornography, keeping in mind that both men and women use pornography for their entertainment and arousal, with pornography and the trauma around it becoming so normalized in our society. Again, just because something is normalized does not mean that it is healthy. The important question we need to ask ourselves through the lens of the fifth mindfulness training is, "Is viewing this nourishing and healing, or is it adding to my trauma?"

A Culture of Nourishment and Healing

It is important to note much that not just pornography is traumatizing and demeaning of our humanity. Much of the media we create and consume, even seemingly "factual" programming, is painful to experience. Just by watching the news, we will inevitably be exposed to dehumanizing, violent images and information. While we must stay aware of current events and not disengage from others' suffering, the unmindful consumption of electronic media has become a source of trauma for our entire society.

How do we cultivate the right conditions for us to thrive, held securely in the arms of our communities, with easy, enjoyable communication between us all? Those of us who have experienced the social life of the past may remember what it used to be like. In Vietnam when I was growing up, it was common for people to wake up early, then sit in a coffee shop or on the sidewalk to have a cup of coffee and talk with friends before going to work. When I was last in Vietnam, in April 2019, I saw people sitting in small coffee shops, and every person was looking down at their iPhone. Nobody made eye contact or talked to anybody else. The lively neighborly back-and-forth conversations had all but disappeared. My heart just dropped. The people were still poor, but now even the sense of community was also stripped from them.

This was no longer the Vietnam I once knew!

Picking me up at the airport, my oldest nephew greeted me sincerely, "Hello, Auntie." Yet the next moment he was already on his iPhone. I hardly ever go back to visit Vietnam, but I found my nephews could not take the initiative to converse with me, or they would make some perfunctory small talk then quickly go back to their phones.

Social isolation is so prevalent now, even though there are still places where interactive human culture still thrives. We have become alienated and distant from nourishing human relationships, and if we don't have human relationships, we can neither experience love nor heal our pain. While the information revolution has undoubtedly changed our world for the better in many ways, we have also become more individualistic, selfish, and lonely. The rate of suicide among young people has increased since the introduction of social media. These are symptoms of societal trauma.

There is a need for collective awareness that our unmindful consumption of electronic media has become a systemic source of new trauma for this generation and generations to come. When we look deeply, we will recognize these dysfunctions in ourselves, our families, and the people we know. Some of us are old enough to remember life before the internet, before AI, before the rise of the large communications companies (aptly called FAANG, like a snake's tooth!*), and we remember when screen-time was less prevalent. We may mourn the past and feel the way we are heading is unhealthy. We can work with this grief to bring mindfulness to our technology use and electronic media consumption. To consciously commit to create a culture that heals and transforms us for the better, as practitioners we are fortunate to have the Five Mindfulness Trainings as a guiding path.

If we have been through some traumatic experiences as children, as teenagers, or as adults, we may feel completely disconnected from our body. This feeling or sensation of disembodiment might have begun as a coping mechanism. When things are extremely stressful at home, or when we are in a situation that is unbearable, our mind can actually "check out," and it can simply hover over and look at the body going through the unpleasant experience; or it can watch an abhorrent event, for example, people battering one another, while having no internal feelings or reactions to the circumstance. This is a way to protect ourselves from feeling the pain or the horror that our body may be going through.

As we grow older and we are no longer in that particular situation, the habit of checking out might have become ingrained in us. It may still be our main coping mechanism every time we feel threatened or pressured or caught in a situation. This is the reality for many of us to a greater or lesser degree. The coping mechanism from our childhood might have saved us then and allowed us to survive, but now it has

---

* FAANG is an acronym referring to the five most popular and powerful American technology companies: Facebook, Amazon, Apple, Netflix, and Google.

become intrusive, either over-sensitizing or numbing every aspect of our lives. This tendency to check out all too easily pairs with addiction to our electronic devices and other aspects of our way of life to cause new levels of isolation, loneliness, and unhealed, unresolved trauma.

Therefore, to counter our unmindful consumption and begin to create a culture of nourishment and healing, it is essential that we learn to heal this sense of disembodiment by establishing equilibrium and coming back to our body. "Breathing in, I am aware that I have a body." "Breathing out, I thank my body. I know you are here, and I'm so grateful." The work seems ever so gentle, but it has powerful effects on us as individuals and collectively. A society made up of people who have healed from trauma is peaceful, nourishing, and safe.

Wherever you are, you can try to sit with stability like a mountain. Smile and send wishes of peace and love to your body. "Thank you, my dear body for being there for me. May I take good care of you. May I choose to be safe and to be happy. May I choose to protect others, so that they too can be happy and safe."

As a nun, I have learned to say a loving mantra to my body frequently throughout the day, "I love you so. Help me to take better care of you." In whichever position I am in—walking, standing, sitting, or lying down—I use the energy of mindfulness to scan through each part of my body, acknowledging it and giving rise to gratitude for what I still have in this moment. It felt strange and awkward to say "I love you" to myself at first, but gradually it has become the most constant and comforting thought and feeling that I carry throughout the day. It has magically replaced and removed self-destructive and self-hating thoughts in me. "I love you" is the most powerful spiritual mantra that we can wield.

CHAPTER 13

Reclaiming Your Power to Heal

Taking refuge in myself.

Coming back to myself.

I am free.

My grandmother never had a chance to go to school. She picked up her first alphabet lessons from her eldest son, who, as a first grader, would teach her how to read from what he had learned at school. Before long, she was able to read and memorize the whole of the legendary Vietnamese epic poem "Tale of Kiều," which has more than three thousand lines.

She could also do arithmetic, all in her head. After my mother disappeared, Grandma started a small shop out of our home, to earn money to raise my brother and me. Every time she purchased some goods, such as firewood bunched together in various sizes, Grandma would always do the math in her head and quickly give out the correct answer of how much to pay, while I was still trying to work out the answer with a pencil and paper! Yet Grandma did not know how to write at all. When a signature was required, with great effort, holding a pen clumsily and tightly in her hand, Grandma would mark an "X" in place of her signature. That X was her signature.

I have been much more fortunate than my grandmother in my educational opportunities. Yet even after twenty-four years of schooling, including medical school, I still deeply feel that I learned most from my grandmother, because she was the one who taught me about love. Even though she wanted to enter monastic life, Grandma could not become a nun, because she had to raise my brother and me in my mother's place. In her rare spare moments, instead of spending time on idle chitchat with neighbors, she would sit still on her plank bed—a wooden bed made of thick, fine hardwood, well-polished by years of use—fingering her prayer beads and softly whispering prayers to the Buddha. The atmosphere in our home would become peaceful and concentrated. I also learned to quiet myself while Grandma was meditating and praying.

On the first night after I had come to Plum Village with the intent to join the monastic life, Grandma appeared in my dream, saying, "In my life I suffered many great afflictions, and I have been able to overcome them all. You will too." I woke up, realizing more clearly than ever that Grandma had always been with me.

Recently, I had an ongoing headache that lasted for a few days. It felt as if a blood vessel on my left temporal region was pulsating with a sharp, sudden jolting pain every few minutes. Besides the discomfort, the jolting aspect was startling, so I did my best to remain mindful of my breath and body, so that I would not be caught by surprise by the pain. I even hesitated to use the restroom, because physically bearing down also triggered jolts of pain.

One morning, after early morning sitting meditation and breakfast, I could not bear the pain any longer, so I went back to bed. I dreamt that I was lying across a large bed, and Grandma was also there. Without words, she signaled me to place my head on her chest. I was afraid that my head was heavy for her fragile chest, but I did it anyway. In my dream, I fell asleep peacefully with my head on Grandma's chest for a long time. When, in my dream, I woke up, she remained still so my head could stay resting on Grandma; I fell asleep again in that position.

When I woke up again close to 10 a.m., my head felt light and free of pain. I went to the bathroom, but there was no pain. I went to the morning's Dharma talk, experiencing two mild pulsations in that left temporal area, and then the pain ceased completely! For the rest of that day, I felt as if the left side of my head was still resting and in contact with my grandmother's chest, which was firm and yet soothing and more comforting than any pillows I had ever experienced. The healing took place in my dream, and it literally ended my headache.

Nothing had been lost! Thirty-five years have passed, and to this day Grandma continues to live within me, guide me, comfort me, and heal me.

In retrospect, the periods of my childhood during which I could live in peace and safety were when I had Grandma living with me. On the other hand, when she was absent—for example, when she remained in the countryside while my mother moved me and my brother to Saigon, to live in the big house with the rich old man and my uncle—these were the times when I suffered from danger and misfortune.

For those of us who have had the opportunity to be an anchor for a young person—as a father, mother, brother, sister, or friend—the biggest present we can offer them is our own presence and our peace. In turn, when we are blessed to have a loved one who is always present for us, either in form or in thought, like Grandma is for me, we'll always have the opportunity to learn and to feel protection, peace, and happiness from that person, even if they are physically no longer present in our lives.

The path of mindfulness allows us to become that loving person for ourselves, as well as for others all around us. I hope that the stories I have shared and the practices in this book will help you to be an island of refuge unto yourself. Through embracing our suffering, developing our capacity to nourish ourselves with the Five Strengths, and training ourselves in the art of mindfulness, we find ourselves amply blessed for healing. We are enough. We have all we need. We simply need to reclaim our power to heal.

I was born in wartime. I came as a sixteen-year-old orphan to the United States, a suitcase in one hand and my brother's hand in the other, sent by our grandmother in search of a peaceful life. During my life there has not been a single year when the planet has been free of conflict between human beings. Yet I know that peace is the birthright of every one of us. Healing from trauma is the way.

Today there are many people in terrible situations, conditions that are bound to create more trauma in the world. We are not only refugees from war, but also refugees from the violence that occurs in our communities and families, even within the walls of seemingly comfortable homes. I know that the conditions for trauma will continue to be created if we do not learn to create the conditions for peace within ourselves and in society. However, I don't despair. I am lucky to live in a community where I see so many people working for peace and for healing, relying on their strengths to generate the energy to overcome whatever negativity may arise. I am so fortunate to have found this path.

Just as we carry the seeds of trauma in us, we also carry the seeds for healing. With trust, diligence, mindfulness, concentration, and insight, we can create the conditions for the flowers of peace to bloom, even in the dark. The world is full of moments of danger, but love is also there all around us, when we look for it and remain steady in ourselves, in our practice, not getting lost in our dramas. The qualities of a bodhisattva are within each one of us, waiting to flower.

Text of the Five Mindfulness Trainings

The text of the Five Mindfulness Trainings can be found on the Plum Village website, plumvillage.org, and are offered below for easy reference.

The Five Mindfulness Trainings have their root in the Five Precepts offered by the Buddha. They have been expanded and updated so that they represent a way to bring mindfulness into every area of life. Rather than hard and fast rules, they offer a framework to reflect on our actions, speech, and thinking, so we can create more happiness for ourselves and for the world around us.

The Five Mindfulness Trainings are one of the most concrete ways to practice mindfulness. They are nonsectarian and universal. They are true practices of compassion and understanding. All spiritual traditions have their equivalent of the Five Mindfulness Trainings.

The first training is to protect life and decrease violence, in oneself, the family, and society. The second training is to practice social justice and generosity, not stealing and not exploiting other living beings. The third is the practice of responsible sexual behavior, in order to protect individuals, couples, families, and children. The fourth is the practice of deep listening and loving speech, to restore communication and reconcile. The fifth is about mindful consumption, to help us not bring toxins and poisons into our body or mind.

The Five Mindfulness Trainings are based on the precepts developed during the time of the Buddha to be the foundation of practice for the entire lay practice community. They are called "mindfulness trainings" because mindfulness is their foundation. With mindfulness, we are aware of what is going on in our bodies, our feelings, our minds, and the world, and we avoid doing harm to ourselves and others. Mindfulness protects us, our families, and our society. When we are mindful, we can see that by refraining from doing one thing, we can prevent another thing from happening. We arrive at our own unique insight. It is not something imposed on us by an outside authority.

Practicing the mindfulness trainings, therefore, helps us to be calmer and more concentrated, and brings more insight and enlightenment.

The Five Mindfulness Trainings

The Five Mindfulness Trainings represent the Buddhist vision for a global spirituality and ethic. They are a concrete expression of the Buddha's teachings on the Four Noble Truths and the Noble Eightfold Path, the path of right understanding and true love, leading to healing, transformation, and happiness for ourselves and for the world. To practice the Five Mindfulness Trainings is to cultivate the insight of interbeing, or Right View, which can remove all discrimination, intolerance, anger, fear, and despair. If we live according to the Five Mindfulness Trainings, we are already on the path of a bodhisattva. Knowing we are on that path, we are not lost in confusion about our life in the present or in fears about the future.

Reverence for Life

Aware of the suffering caused by the destruction of life, I am committed to cultivating the insight of interbeing and compassion and learning ways to protect the lives of people, animals, plants, and minerals. I am determined not to kill, not to let others kill, and not to support any act of killing in the world, in my thinking, or in my way of life. Seeing that harmful actions arise from anger, fear, greed, and intolerance, which in turn come from dualistic and discriminative thinking, I will cultivate openness, non-discrimination, and non-attachment to views in order to transform violence, fanaticism, and dogmatism in myself and in the world.

True Happiness

Aware of the suffering caused by exploitation, social injustice, stealing, and oppression, I am committed to practicing generosity in my thinking, speaking, and acting. I am determined not to steal and not to possess anything that should belong to others; and I will share my time, energy, and material resources with those who are in need. I will practice looking deeply to see that the happiness and suffering of others are not separate from my own happiness and suffering; that true happiness is not possible without understanding and compassion; and that running after wealth, fame, power, and sensual pleasures can bring much suffering and despair. I am aware that happiness depends on my mental attitude and not on external conditions, and that I can live happily in the present moment simply by remembering that I already have more than enough conditions to be happy. I am committed to practicing Right Livelihood so that I can help reduce the suffering of living beings on Earth and stop contributing to climate change.

True Love

Aware of the suffering caused by sexual misconduct, I am committed to cultivating responsibility and learning ways to protect the safety and integrity of individuals, couples, families, and society. Knowing that sexual desire is not love, and that sexual activity motivated by craving always harms myself as well as others, I am determined not to engage in sexual relations without true love and a deep, long-term commitment made known to my family and friends. I will do everything in my power to protect children from sexual abuse and to prevent couples and families from being broken by sexual misconduct. Seeing that body and mind are one, I am committed to learning appropriate ways to take care of my sexual energy and cultivating loving kindness, compassion, joy, and inclusiveness—which are the four basic elements of true love—for my greater happiness and the greater happiness of others. Practicing true love, we know that we will continue beautifully into the future.

Loving Speech and Deep Listening

Aware of the suffering caused by unmindful speech and the inability to listen to others, I am committed to cultivating loving speech and compassionate listening in order to relieve suffering and to promote reconciliation and peace in myself and among other people, ethnic and religious groups, and nations. Knowing that words can create happiness or suffering, I am committed to speaking truthfully using words that inspire confidence, joy, and hope. When anger is manifesting in me, I am determined not to speak. I will practice mindful breathing and walking in order to recognize and to look deeply into my anger. I know that the roots of anger can be found in my wrong perceptions and lack of understanding of the suffering in myself and in the other person. I will speak and listen in a way that can help myself and the other person to transform suffering and see the way out of difficult situations. I am determined not to spread news that I do not know to be certain and not to utter words that can cause division or discord. I will practice Right Diligence to nourish my capacity for understanding, love, joy, and inclusiveness, and gradually transform anger, violence, and fear that lie deep in my consciousness.

Nourishment and Healing

Aware of the suffering caused by unmindful consumption, I am committed to cultivating good health, both physical and mental, for myself, my family, and my society by practicing mindful eating, drinking, and consuming. I will practice looking deeply into how I consume the Four Kinds of Nutriments, namely edible foods, sense impressions, volition, and consciousness. I am determined not to gamble, or to use alcohol, drugs, or any other products which contain toxins, such as certain websites, electronic games, TV programs, films, magazines, books, and conversations. I will practice coming back to the present moment to be in touch with the refreshing, healing, and nourishing elements in me and around me, not letting regrets and sorrow drag me back into the past nor letting anxieties, fear, or craving pull me out of the present moment. I am determined not to try to cover up loneliness, anxiety, or other suffering by losing myself in consumption. I will contemplate interbeing and consume in a way that preserves peace, joy, and well-being in my body and consciousness, and in the collective body and consciousness of my family, my society, and the Earth.

COMMUNITIES FOR MINDFULNESS, HEALING, AND TRANSFORMATION

The Plum Village Community of Engaged Buddhism: *plumvillage.org*

Deer Park Monastery: *deerparkmonastery.org*

To find a local group with whom to practice mindfulness and the path of healing and transformation, see the global Plum Village Sangha Directory: *www.plumline.org/directory*

COMMUNITIES FOR TRAUMA HEALING

RAINN (Rape, Abuse and Incest National Network) is the United States's largest anti-sexual violence organization. RAINN created and operates the National Sexual Assault Hotline (800.656.HOPE) in partnership with more than 1,000 local sexual assault service providers across the country. Get help 24/7. *RAINN.org*

Somatic Experiencing: *traumahealing.org*

Trauma Resource Institute: *traumaresourceinstitute.com*

MINDFULNESS BELLS

The Plum Village App has beautiful bell recordings from Plum Village Monastery, which you may set at intervals to remind you to stop and breathe as you go through your day: *plumvillage.app*

BOOKS BY THICH NHAT HANH

Nhat Hanh, Thich. *The Blooming of a Lotus: Revised Edition of the Classic Guided Meditation for Achieving the Miracle of Mindfulness.* Boston: Beacon Press, 2009.

———. *Breathe! You Are Alive: Sutra on the Full Awareness of Breathing.* Berkeley, CA: Parallax Press, 1996.

———. *Chanting from the Heart: Buddhist Ceremonies and Daily Practices.* Berkeley, CA: Parallax Press, 2002.

———. *Happiness: Essential Mindfulness Practices.* Berkeley, CA: Parallax Press, 2005.

———. *The Heart of the Buddha's Teaching: Transforming Suffering into Peace, Joy, and Liberation.* New York: Harmony Books, 1999.

———. *How to Eat.* Berkeley, CA: Parallax Press, 2014.

———. *The Mindfulness Survival Kit: Five Essential Practices.* Berkeley, CA: Parallax Press, YEAR.

———. *The Miracle of Mindfulness.* Boston: Beacon Press, 1996.

———. *Reconciliation: Healing the Inner Child.* Berkeley, CA: Parallax Press, 2006.

——— and Cheung, Lilian. *Savor: Mindful Eating, Mindful Life.* San Francisco: HarperOne, 2011.

———. *Touching the Earth: Guided Meditations for Mindfulness Practice.* Berkeley: Parallax Press, 2004.

BOOKS ON TRAUMA AND HEALING

Burke-Harris, Nadine. *The Deepest Well: Healing the Long-Term Effects of Childhood Adversity.* Houghton Mifflin Harcourt, 2018.

Chan Khong, Sister. *Beginning Anew: Four Steps to Restoring Communication.* Berkeley, CA: Parallax Press, 2014.

Dang Nghiem, Sister. *Healing: A Woman's Journey from Doctor to Nun.* Berkeley, CA: Parallax Press, 2010.

———. *Mindfulness as Medicine: A Story of Healing Body and Spirit.* Berkeley, CA: Parallax Press, 2015.

Erikson, Erik. *Childhood and Society.* New York: W. W. Norton, 1950.

Hanson, Rick. *Buddha's Brain* The Practical Neuroscience of Happiness, Love and Wisdom. Oakland, CA: New Harbinger, 2014.

Herman, Judith L. *Trauma and Recovery: The Aftermath of Violence—From Domestic Abuse to Political Terror.* New York: Basic Books, 2015.

LaPierre, Aline, and Laurence Heller. *Healing Developmental Trauma: How Early Trauma Affects Self-Regulation, Self-Image, and the Capacity for Relationship.* Berkeley, CA: North Atlantic Books, 2012.

Levine, Peter A. *Waking the Tiger, Healing Trauma.* Berkeley, CA: North Atlantic Books, 1997.

Simmons, Aisha, ed. *Love with Accountability: Digging up the Roots of Child Sexual Abuse.* Chico, CA: AK Press, 2020.

Siegel, Daniel J. *The Developing Mind, Third Edition: How Relationships and the Brain Interact to Shape Who We Are.* New York: The Guilford Press, 2020.

Stevenson, Bryan. *Just Mercy: A Story of Justice and Redemption.* New York: One World, 2015.

Van der Kolk, Bessel. *The Body Keeps the Score: Brain, Mind, and Body in the Healing of Trauma.* New York: Penguin, 2015.

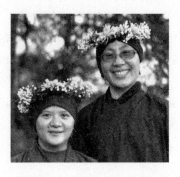

ACKNOWLEDGMENTS

I express my deepest gratitude to our beloved teacher, Zen Master Thich Nhat Hanh. Thanks to Thay's love and wisdom, I may have a path of peace, joy, and no regret.

To my beloved Grandmother, who continues to be a beacon of love in my life.

To my beloved community of Sisters and Brothers at our monasteries all over the world who have grown up with me on the Path.

My deep gratitude to Sister Trúc Nghiêm (aka Sister Bamboo), Sister Thần Nghiêm, Sister Trú Nghiêm for your sisterhood, love, and enduring support.

To my editor, Hisae Matsuda. Thank you for believing in me and in this book, and for making it a reality. Thank you to the staff of Parallax Press for your dedication.

To Cyrus Maher, Lisa Lee, Teja Watson, Katie Eberle, Howie Severson, and Jessica Sevey for your incredible support.

To all the friends who have trusted your stories with me. May our voices help bring understanding and healing in the world.

To all young people, including my niece, Sunee-Hương Trà. May you always be safe and fully blossom into healers and Great Beings.

In honor of all brothers and sisters who have suffered from trauma and abuse. May you find the path. May you flower beautifully into your own magnificence.

I wrote this poem for walking in the rain, which reminds me of John, my beloved partner. With each line, I take a breath and I take a step or two. As I walk, I find myself becoming filled with appreciation for being alive.

> *This morning I walk,*
> Raindrops follow my footsteps.
> Each drop of rain
> Deepens my gratitude
> for you,
> for life.

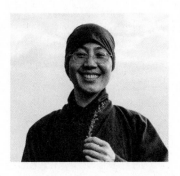

ABOUT SISTER DANG NGHIEM, MD

Sister Dang Nghiem was born in 1968 in Vietnam during the Tet Offensive, the daughter of a Vietnamese mother and an American soldier. She lost her mother at the age of twelve and immigrated to the United States at the age of sixteen with her brother. Living in various foster homes, she learned English and went on to earn a medical degree from the University of California, San Francisco School of Medicine. After suffering further tragedy and loss, she gave up her practice as a doctor to travel to Plum Village monastery in France founded by Zen Master Thich Nhat Hanh, where she was ordained a nun in 2000. She was appointed a Dharma teacher by Thich Nhat Hanh in 2008. She is the author of two books: a memoir, *Healing: A Woman's Journey from Doctor to Nun* (2010), and *Mindfulness as Medicine: A Story of Healing and Spirit* (2015).

OTHER BOOKS FROM PARALLAX PRESS

THICH NHAT HANH

Happiness

The Mindfulness Survival Kit: Five Essential Practices

Reconciliation

SISTER CHAN KHONG

Beginning Anew

SISTER DANG NGHIEM, MD

Healing: A Woman's Journey from Doctor to Nun

Mindfulness as Medicine: A Story of Healing and Spirit

SAEEDA HAFIZ

The Healing: One Woman's Journey from Poverty to Inner Riches

DANIEL JIN BLUM

Sleep Wise: How to Feel Better, Work Smarter, and Build Resilience

ROBERT LESOINE AND MARILYNNE CHOPHEL

Unfinished Conversation: Healing from Suicide and Loss

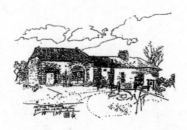

Monastics and visitors practice the art of mindful living in the tradition of Thich Nhat Hanh at our mindfulness practice centers around the world. To reach any of these communities, or for information about how individuals, couples, and families can join in a retreat, please contact:

PLUM VILLAGE
33580 Dieulivol, France
plumvillage.org

MAGNOLIA GROVE MONASTERY
Batesville, MS 38606, USA
magnoliagrovemonastery.org

BLUE CLIFF MONASTERY
Pine Bush, NY 12566, USA
bluecliffmonastery.org

DEER PARK MONASTERY
Escondido, CA 92026, USA
deerparkmonastery.org

EUROPEAN INSTITUTE OF
APPLIED BUDDHISM
D-51545 Waldbröl, Germany
eiab.eu

THAILAND PLUM VILLAGE
Nakhon Ratchasima
30130 Thailand
thaiplumvillage.org

ASIAN INSTITUTE OF
APPLIED BUDDHISM
Lantau Island, Hong Kong
pvfhk.org

LA MAISON DE L'INSPIR
77510 Verdelot, France
maisondelinspir.org

HEALING SPRING MONASTERY
77510 Verdelot, France
healingspringmonastery.org

STREAM ENTERING MONASTERY
Beaufort, Victoria 3373, Australia
nhapluu.org

The Mindfulness Bell, a journal of the art of mindful living in the tradition of Thich Nhat Hanh, is published three times a year by our community. To subscribe or to see the worldwide directory of Sanghas, or local mindfulness groups, visit mindfulnessbell.org.

PARALLAX PRESS, a nonprofit publisher founded by Zen Master Thich Nhat Hanh, publishes books and media on the art of mindful living and Engaged Buddhism. We are committed to offering teachings that help transform suffering and injustice. Our aspiration is to contribute to collective insight and awakening, bringing about a more joyful, healthy, and compassionate society.

View our entire library at parallax.org.